Practice Papers for MCEM Part A

Practice Papers for MCEM Part A

Jaydeep Chitnis, MBBS, FEM (India), MRCS (Ed)
Specialist Registrar in Emergency Medicine
Emergency Department
Southampton General Hospital
Southampton, UK

Gary Cumberbatch, FRCS (Ed), DA (UK), FCEM
Consultant in Emergency Medicine
Emergency Department
Poole Hospital
Poole, UK

Ananda U H Gankande, FRCS (Ed)
Associate Specialist
Emergency Department
Poole Hospital NHS Foundation Trust
Longfleet Road
Poole, UK

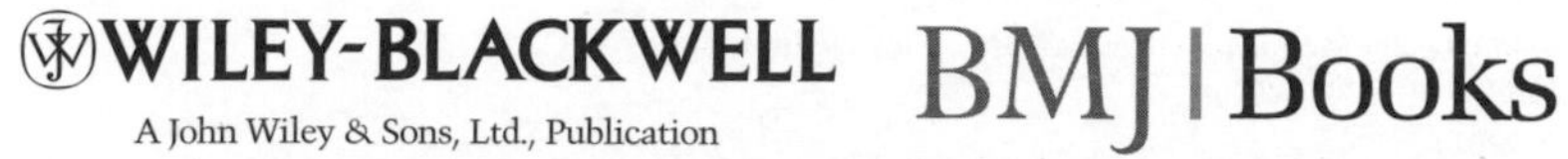

BMJ Books is an imprint of BMJ Publishing Group Limited, used under licence by Blackwell Publishing which was acquired by John Wiley & Sons in February 2007. Blackwell's publishing programme has been merged with Wiley's global Scientific, Technical and Medical business to form Wiley-Blackwell.

Registered office: John Wiley & Sons Ltd, The Atrium, Southern Gate, Chichester, West Sussex, PO19 8SQ, UK

Editorial offices: 9600 Garsington Road, Oxford, OX4 2DQ, UK
The Atrium, Southern Gate, Chichester, West Sussex, PO19 8SQ, UK
111 River Street, Hoboken, NJ 07030-5774, USA

For details of our global editorial offices, for customer services and for information about how to apply for permission to reuse the copyright material in this book please see our website at www.wiley.com/wiley-blackwell

Library of Congress Cataloging-in-Publication Data

Chitnis, Jaydeep.
Practice papers for MCEM part A / Jaydeep Chitnis, Gary Cumberpatch, Ananda U.H. Gankande.
p. ; cm.
ISBN 978-1-4443-3068-7 (pbk. : alk. paper)
1. Emergency medicine–Examinations, questions, etc. I. Cumberpatch, Gary.
II. Gankande, Ananda U. H. III. Title.
[DNLM: 1. Emergencies–Examination Questions. 2. Emergency Medicine–Examination Questions. WB 18.2 C543p 2010]
RC86.7.C47 2010
616.02′5076–dc22

2009031392

ISBN: 978-1-4443-3068-7

A catalogue record for this book is available from the British Library.

Set in 9/12pt Meridien by Aptara® Inc., New Delhi, India
Printed in Singapore

2 2011

Contents

Preface

The Membership of the College of Emergency Medicine examination was first held in 2003 (initially known as MFAEM). It is now a prerequisite to pass this examination before undertaking higher training in emergency medicine. There is a dearth of practice questions and papers specifically targeted at the MCEM-A examination. We have put together 8 practice papers (altogether 400 questions) along with answers for the MCEM part-A examination. These are based on the syllabus of the College of Emergency Medicine and each subject area has been given the appropriate proportion according to the College examination guidance. We hope that this book will be helpful for candidates preparing for this examination by identifying knowledge deficiencies and quickly correcting them through the succinct answers provided.

We would like to thank all members of our respective families for their support and patience during the time of writing this book.

Jaydeep Chitnis
Gary Cumberbatch
Upali Gankande

November 2009

Practice Papers

Practice Paper 1

1 Regarding the portal venous system

a) The portal vein is formed by the union of the splenic vein and the superior mesenteric vein

b) The inferior mesenteric vein drains blood from the ascending and transverse colon

c) Elevated portal venous pressure causes caput medusae

d) Right and left gastric veins draining the lesser curve of the stomach are tributaries to the left hepatic vein

2 In the skull

a) The frontal bone articulates with the parietal bone at the lambdoid suture

b) The facial nerve passes through the stylomastoid foramen

c) The zygomatic arch is formed by the zygomatic processes of the frontal and temporal bones

d) The optic nerve passes through the superior orbital fissure

3 Regarding pain

a) In the dorsal columns, sensory signals are carried in small nerve fibres

b) The thalamus has a role in determining the type of sensation a person feels

c) Pain elicits an immediate high level of excitability in the brainstem and cerebrum which can manifest itself in screaming

d) One pain control mechanism is by transmitting signals from the cerebrum to the posterior horns of the spinal cord to inhibit transmission of pain

4 The cardiac output increases with

a) Moderate changes in environmental temperature

b) Standing from a lying down position

c) Eating

d) Rapid arrhythmias

5 Thiopentone sodium

a) Is a barbiturate and is dissolved in normal saline
b) Reduces cerebral metabolic rate, cerebral blood flow and intracranial pressure
c) Is highly protein bound
d) May damage nerves and cause tissue necrosis if it extravasates

6 Aspirin can cause asthma in a sensitive person by

a) Releasing histamine from mast cells
b) Increasing the formation of leukotriene D4 in the lungs
c) Its beta-adrenoceptor blocking action
d) Increasing renal clearance of endogenous noradrenalin

7 The following are brainstem reflexes

a) The knee-jerk reflex
b) The oculocephalic reflex
c) The vestibulocochlear reflex
d) The pupillary reflex

8 Plasma renin activity is most likely to be decreased in

a) Gram-negative shock
b) Haemorrhagic shock
c) Standing quietly
d) Essential hypertension

9 The vertebral column

a) Is made up of 33 vertebrae
b) Has intervertebral foramina which are formed by notches in the laminae
c) Has C1 to C7 segmental spinal nerves passing over the superior aspect of their corresponding vertebrae
d) Results in spina bifida if the two primary ossification centres of the body do not fuse

10 The mitral valve

a) Cusps are avascular
b) Has no papillary muscle attachments
c) Has a larger posterior cusp which lies between the aortic and mitral orifices
d) 'Guards' the right atrioventricular orifice

11 Regarding study design
- **a)** Hypothesis is a prediction
- **b)** In a cross-over study each patient receives treatment and placebo in a random order
- **c)** Case–control study is a type of observational study
- **d)** Blinding reduces bias in treatment studies

12 Regarding the red blood cell
- **a)** The diameter of the biconcave erythrocyte is more than that of the capillaries
- **b)** Haemoglobin makes up about 30% of the dry weight of the red blood cell
- **c)** Adult haemoglobin A1 has lower affinity for oxygen than foetal haemoglobin
- **d)** Red blood cells carry 10 times the amount of oxygen that can be carried in plasma alone

13 In the unconscious patient
- **a)** Vomiting can occur at any time
- **b)** The administration of naloxone should always be considered when the diagnosis is uncertain
- **c)** They should always be transferred to a high-dependency area once stable
- **d)** A CT scan of the head is required

14 While working in an emergency department
- **a)** Make concise notes
- **b)** The allocated triage category for a patient may change with time
- **c)** You can provide a written police statement without patient consent
- **d)** Do not delay life-saving treatment in order to obtain consent

15 The tongue
- **a)** Has no papillae over its posterior half
- **b)** In its anterior 2/3 receives its sensory supply from the trigeminal nerve
- **c)** Has all its muscles supplied by the hypoglossal nerve
- **d)** Can be brought off the posterior pharyngeal wall of the unconscious patient by using the jaw thrust because it is attached to the symphysis of the mandible by genioglossus

16 The diaphragm

a) Has an opening at the level of T10 through which the aorta and thoracic duct are transmitted

b) Transmits the inferior vena cava through its muscular portion at T8

c) In its central part receives sensory fibres that run in the phrenic nerve

d) When paralysed is recognised radiographically by its flattening and paradoxical movements

17 Tuberculosis

a) Can remain dormant for years

b) Can present atypically in immunocompromised patients

c) Can be excluded in a symptomatic patient if the chest X-ray is normal

d) If suspected in a patient in the ED, the patient should be isolated

18 Pelvic inflammatory disease

a) Includes salpingitis

b) There is a 5% increased risk of ectopic pregnancy as a sequelae

c) Causative organisms include *Chlamydia trachomatis* and *Mycoplasma hominis*

d) May be symptom-free

19 Drug antagonism

a) Can occur with pharmacokinetic interference

b) May be potentially irreversible

c) Can occur with chemical antagonism

d) Can occur as a result of interaction with receptor sites

20 Which of the following statements are true

a) Phenytoin when given to a patient on warfarin will reduce the plasma concentration of the latter

b) Calcium-channel blockers decrease the plasma concentration of midazolam but increase the concentration of digoxin in the plasma

c) Cimetidine is a P450 enzyme activator

d) Labetolol (beta-blocker) plasma concentration is decreased by the concomitant use of cimetidine

21 Regarding water and electrolytes
- **a)** Insensible water loss can be between 500 and 850 mL/day
- **b)** A rise in intracellular osmolality inhibits the secretion of antidiuretic hormone
- **c)** Aldosterone increases urinary sodium excretion
- **d)** The juxtaglomerular apparatus secretes renin in response to high blood pressure

22 An ECG showing ST segment elevation may be
- **a)** From an athlete
- **b)** Due to hypokalaemia
- **c)** Due to a sternal fracture sustained in a road traffic collision
- **d)** As a result of systolic load

23 Regarding clinical symptoms and signs
- **a)** Anaphylaxis may present with swelling of lips and tongue with wheezing
- **b)** Cholecystitis may present with chest pain
- **c)** History and clinical examination can always safely exclude a deep vein thrombosis
- **d)** Brushing of hair induces severe pain in trigeminal neuralgia

24 In patients with burns
- **a)** The adult head covers 9% of the total body surface area
- **b)** Drooling or dribbling of saliva can suggest smoke inhalation
- **c)** Full thickness burns are very painful
- **d)** In chemical burns, acids are more destructive and penetrate more deeply than alkalis

25 The following is true in anaemias
- **a)** Aplastic anaemia can be caused by an idiosyncratic reaction to chloramphenicol ingestion
- **b)** Fanconi's anaemia is a type of megaloblastic anaemia
- **c)** Subleukaemic leukaemia commonly presents with pancytopenia
- **d)** A microcytic hypochromic anaemia is seen in β-thalassaemia

26 The following is true in infectious mononucleosis
- **a)** It usually spreads in an epidemic
- **b)** Splenomegaly occurs in less than 10% of cases

c) Atypical lymphocytosis is a characteristic finding
d) Differential diagnosis includes acute cytomegalovirus infection and toxoplasmosis

27 The hip joint
a) Is abducted by gluteus medius and minimus
b) Is innervated by two nerves: the sciatic nerve and the femoral nerve
c) Is the largest joint in the body
d) Can dislocate posteriorly, anteriorly and centrally

28 The cerebellum
a) Has its cortex made up of grey matter
b) Has the dentate nucleus within the centre of each hemisphere
c) Contributes to the posterior wall of the IVth ventricle
d) If pathologically affected can result in nystagmus and dysarthria

29 The uterus
a) Is crossed laterally above its middle by the ureter
b) Is supported by the anterior cardinal ligaments
c) Is related posteriorly to the uterovesical pouch
d) Derives its entire blood supply from the uterine arteries

30 The following is true in normal distribution
a) It is symmetric and bell-shaped
b) The mean, median and mode may have the same value
c) 90% of the values will lie between two standard deviations from the mean
d) The median is the best measure of central tendency

31 Regarding the immune system
a) B lymphocytes are essential for humoral immunity
b) About 60–70% of lymphocytes in the blood are B lymphocytes
c) IgM is the most abundant of circulating immunoglobulins
d) IgG is the only immunoglobulin that crosses the placenta

32 All of the following are antidotes for the corresponding drugs taken in overdose
a) Sodium nitrate for cyanide poisoning
b) Desferrioxamine for iron poisoning
c) Calcium gluconate gel for hydrochloric acid burns
d) IV ethanol for ethylene glycol poisoning

33 Nitrous oxide

a) Is predominantly excreted by exhalation
b) Increases blood pressure and heart rate
c) During recovery, transient hypoxia may occur in patients with respiratory disease
d) Is a powerful muscle relaxant

34 Thyroxine

a) Is formed by elemental iodine and thyroglobulin
b) Is rapidly released into tissues to enable an immediate metabolic response to stress
c) Is thought to increase the number of intracellular enzymes and hence increase the rate of metabolism of cells
d) Can increase the body's metabolic rate by 10-fold

35 Regarding surface anatomy in the upper limb

a) The ulnar nerve passes behind the lateral epicondyle of the humerus
b) The extensor pollicis longus forms the lateral border of the anatomical snuff box
c) The pisiform bone is easily palpable at the distal end of the flexor carpi ulnaris tendon
d) The cubital fossa contains the brachial artery and the median nerve

36 In an AP X-ray of the pelvis

a) Ossification of cartilage at the junction of the ischial and pubic bones can be mistaken for a fracture in a child
b) The symphysis pubis is usually wider than 5 mm in an adult
c) A double break in a 'ring' is an unstable injury
d) A fracture at one point in the 'ring' is not associated frequently with a second fracture in the 'ring'

37 Regarding the JVP

a) Prominent 'a' waves occur in atrial fibrillation
b) Giant 'v' waves are seen in tricuspid stenosis
c) Kusmaul's sign is indicative of right ventricular infarction
d) 'a' waves occur with ventricular systole

38 To maintain the body in an upright position

a) Antigravity reflexes are integrated in the midbrain
b) Tonic labyrinthine reflexes play an important role

c) Proprioception in distal flexors causes a negative supporting reaction
d) Neck proprioceptors are the receptors for the tonic neck reflexes

39 Addison's disease
a) Has many causes including simple atrophy, prolonged excessive overstimulation and Friderichsen–Waterhouse syndrome
b) Can cause death in just a few days due to severe extracellular fluid volume depletion
c) Can be easily treated by daily ingestion of a large dose of mineralocorticoids
d) Also requires a patient to need to take a glucocorticoid to be able to mount an adequate stress response

40 Tetanus
a) 15–25% of patients may not have evidence of recent wounds
b) Prone wounds include superficial burns and crush injuries
c) Endotoxin causes muscle spasm and rigidity
d) Prevention in a patient at high risk includes human tetanus immunoglobulin given IM

41 Myocarditis
a) May be caused by diphtheria or trypanosomiasis
b) Can be due to a viral infection, typically paramyxovirus
c) Often causes acute left ventricular failure
d) Generally has a good prognosis

42 The long saphenous vein
a) Drains directly into the femoral vein just below the inguinal ligament
b) Communicates with the deep veins via a multitude of perforating veins
c) Has two large tributaries which drain into it at the level of the groin
d) Is situated just anterior and superior to the medial malleolus

43 Regarding the skin
a) The cutaneous nerves have efferent somatic fibres and afferent autonomic fibres
b) The nails grow faster in immobilised limbs than normally

c) Boils and carbuncles start in hair follicles and sebaceous glands
d) The stratum corneum of the epidermis is made up of dead cells without any nuclei

44 Regarding leukaemoid reactions
a) May be either myeloid or lymphoid
b) Proportion of immature cells is usually very high
c) Marrow aspiration and trephine biopsy is needed to differentiate from leukaemia
d) Can be seen in acute haemolytic anaemia

45 The following can cause petechiae or ecchymoses
a) Uraemia
b) Furosemide
c) Typhoid fever
d) Cryoglobulinaemia

46 Events that occur in wound healing include
a) Cell mutation
b) Neovascularisation
c) Inhibition of growth factors
d) Chemotaxis

47 The following arterial blood gas was obtained from an ill patient in the resuscitation room who was on 15 L/min of oxygen: pH $= 7.10$, $PaCO_2 = 3.9$ KPa, $PaO_2 = 40$ KPa, $HCO_3 = 12$ mmol/L, BE $= -12$, $K^+ = 6.0$ mmol/L, $Na^+ = 145$ mmol/L, $Cl^- = 98$ mmol/L
a) The patient has a metabolic acidosis with an anion gap of 31
b) The elevated potassium could be simply attributed to the metabolic acidosis
c) The patient is making little respiratory compensation
d) All of the following could be potential causes: diabetic ketoacidosis, ethylene glycol poisoning, cyanide poisoning or the postictal state

48 In respiratory pathology
a) Foreign body aspiration causes obstructive atelectasis
b) Recurrent pulmonary emboli cause pulmonary hypertension
c) Tension pneumothorax improves venous return
d) α1-antitrypsin deficiency leads to emphysema

49 In chronic renal failure
- **a)** Erythropoietin deficiency causes hypochromic microcytic anaemia
- **b)** Secondary hyperparathyroidism causes renal osteodystrophy
- **c)** Dietary sodium restriction may be required to prevent sodium overload
- **d)** No symptoms may develop till glomerular filtration rate falls below 10% of normal

50 Regarding herd immunity
- **a)** Herd immunity does not apply to all diseases
- **b)** It is affected by environmental factors such as overcrowding
- **c)** Non-immunised people are protected due to herd immunity
- **d)** Herd immunity is more effective as the percentage of people vaccinated increases

Practice Paper 2

1 The following are signs and symptoms of hypercapnoea

a) Headache
b) Drowsiness
c) Dry pale skin
d) Conjunctival congestion

2 Respiratory infections in children

a) Acute laryngotracheobronchitis is caused by parainfluenza viruses in 75% of cases
b) In acute epiglottitis, a thorough examination of the throat should be performed immediately
c) The peak incidence of acute bronchiolitis is between 3 and 6 years
d) Acute epiglottitis is usually caused by the respiratory syncytial virus and does not require antibiotic therapy

3 The ulnar nerve

a) Passes deep to the flexor retinaculum and lies lateral to the pisiform bone
b) Supplies the adductor pollicis muscle
c) Lies medial to the flexor carpi ulnaris tendon at the wrist
d) Injury at the level of wrist results in clawing which is most pronounced in index and middle fingers

4 Regarding visceral innervation in the abdomen

a) The myenteric and submucosal plexuses coordinate gastric secretory activity and peristalsis
b) Parasympathetic innervation to the gastrointestinal system is solely from the vagus nerve
c) Referred pain from midgut organs is felt in the flanks and pubic region
d) The celiac and superior mesenteric ganglia are associated with the abdominal prevertebral plexus

5 When reading a paper offering clinical evidence

a) A *p* value of less than 1 in 20 is considered 'statistically significant'

b) The standard error of mean is smaller for larger sample sizes

c) Pseudo-randomisation does not allow pure chance to match the subjects to the groups

d) Blinding of patients to the treatment reduces the bias introduced by the placebo effect

6 Regarding formation of blood cells

a) Production of blood cells commences in the yolk sac of the embryo

b) Extramedullary haemopoiesis occurs in the liver and spleen

c) The mature red cell is slightly greater in volume and diameter than the reticulocyte

d) The approximate lifespan of the red blood cell is 120 days

7 You can end your professional relationship with a patient if

a) The patient has been violent to you

b) The patient has been violent to your colleague

c) The patient has stolen from the premises

d) The patient has made a complaint about you or your team

8 The criteria for diagnosis of SIRS (systemic inflammatory response syndrome) are

a) Blood pressure <90 mm Hg systolic

b) Temperature >38°C or <36°C

c) WBC count $<4000/mm^3$ or $>12,000/mm^3$

d) Elevated CRP

9 The following are true of the hypothalamus

a) It forms the roof of the third ventricle

b) Is mainly concerned with autonomic function

c) It includes the optic chiasma, the tuber cinereum and the mamillary bodies

d) A lesion here can result in somnolence and obesity

10 The symphysis pubis

a) Is a primary cartilaginous joint

b) Is lined with synovial membrane

c) Is separated in an 'open book' type pelvis fracture

d) Is strengthened inferiorly by the arcuate pubic ligament

11 The following is true in candidiasis

a) Candida albicans are part of the normal flora of the skin

b) Chronic mucocutaneous candidiasis is associated with B-cell lymphocyte dysfunction

c) Candida pneumonia presents most commonly as bronchopneumonia

d) Lactobacillus acidophilus prevent yeast overgrowth and pathogenic infection with candida

12 The following are used in chemoprophylaxis for contacts of meningococcal meningitis

a) Rifampicin

b) Ceftriaxone

c) Ciprofloxacin

d) Flucloxacillin

13 Regarding anticonvulsants

a) Carbamazepine decreases the clearance of other antiepileptic drugs

b) Sodium valproate has its effect by blocking sodium channels

c) Diplopia and ataxia are the most common side effects of phenobarbitone

d) Hirsutism is a rare side effect of phenytoin

14 Regarding antibiotics

a) They principally act by either inhibiting bacterial cell wall synthesis or altering cell wall permeability

b) The difference in susceptibility of Gram-positive and Gram-negative bacteria depends on structural differences in their cell walls

c) β-lactam antibiotics are all inactivated when they are exposed to bacteria which produce β-lactamase lytic enzymes

d) Tetracyclines act by altering the permeability of the cytoplasmic membrane of bacteria so nucleotides, proteins and ions escape resulting in cell death

15 The heart rate is slowed by

a) Stimulation of pain fibres in the trigeminal nerve

b) The increased activities of baroreceptors in the pulmonary circulation

c) Raised intracranial pressure

d) Increased activity of atrial stretch receptors

16 Bone

a) Matrix is mostly type II collagen
b) Osteoblasts are inhibited by glucocorticoids
c) Rapidly takes up lead and isotopes from the body
d) Has a pool of over 25,000 mmols of readily exchangeable calcium

17 In the unconscious patient

a) The principles of management are different for a child
b) Intubation is always needed to protect the airway from gastric aspiration
c) Hypotension can be caused by severely elevated intracranial pressure
d) A bedside glucose measurement should be the first blood test done

18 Regarding the brachial plexus

a) Severe trauma to the first rib usually affects the roots of the brachial plexus
b) Dislocation of shoulder joint can cause injury to the divisions and cords of the brachial plexus
c) Following a nerve avulsion in brachial plexus injury, return of function can usually be expected in 3 weeks of dedicated rehabilitation
d) A brachial plexus nerve block does not block sensation on the dorsum of the forearm

19 Regarding the white cells

a) Lymphocytes are produced in the bone marrow as well as in the lymph nodes
b) The blood neutrophil count represents only about half the total number of neutrophils in the vascular compartment
c) Normal white cell count in childhood tends to be greater than in adults
d) Overwhelming infection leads to a fall in the neutrophil count

20 The following is true in platelet disorders

a) The platelet count is $<100 \times 10^9/L$ in thrombasthenia
b) Thrombocytosis is seen in non-infective inflammatory disorders
c) Chronic idiopathic thrombocytopenic purpura is most commonly a disease of young to middle-aged females
d) There is a 100% response rate to splenectomy in chronic idiopathic thrombocytopenic purpura if steroid therapy has failed

21 The popliteal artery
- **a)** Is deep to both the popliteal vein and tibial nerve
- **b)** Divides at the upper border of the popliteus muscle
- **c)** Is commonly injured in posterior dislocation of the knee joint
- **d)** Is easily palpable

22 With regards to the coronary arteries
- **a)** They arise from within the sinuses of Valsalva
- **b)** In 85–90% of cases, the posterior interventricular artery is a branch of the left coronary artery
- **c)** The SA node is supplied by the right coronary artery in less than 10% of the population
- **d)** The acute marginal branch arises from the left coronary artery

23 The spinal cord
- **a)** Occupies the entire vertebral canal at birth
- **b)** Finishes at the level of the bottom of L2 in the adult
- **c)** Is ensheathed by pia mater which continues inferiorly as the filum terminale and becomes attached to the sacrum
- **d)** Lumbar puncture can be safely performed through the intervertebral disc spaces which lie immediately above and below a line drawn between the iliac crests

24 Consider the following results from a diagnosis study

		Target Disorder	
		Present	Absent
Diagnostic test	Positive	90	5
	Negative	10	105

- **a)** Sensitivity = 85%
- **b)** Specificity = 90%
- **c)** Likelihood ratio for a positive test result = 18
- **d)** Likelihood ratio for a negative test result = 0.10

25 A wound
- **a)** Is a break in the epithelial integrity of the skin
- **b)** May result from a haematoma
- **c)** Heals by primary healing in 3–4 days
- **d)** Showing excessive healing may result in a keloid scar

26 The half-life of a drug
- **a)** Is the time required to change the amount of drug in the body by one-half during elimination
- **b)** Depends solely on the volume of distribution of the drug
- **c)** Depends on both the volume of distribution and the clearance of the drug
- **d)** Disease states can affect the half-life of a drug

27 The following may induce bronchospasm in asthmatics
- **a)** Atropine
- **b)** Aspirin
- **c)** Histamine
- **d)** Propanolol

28 In diabetic ketoacidosis
- **a)** The whole body potassium is normal to high
- **b)** It is a high anion gap acidosis
- **c)** The severe metabolic acidosis is made worse by the increased respiratory rate
- **d)** The insulin dose requirements are lower than in hyperosmolar non-ketotic coma

29 In the shoulder girdle
- **a)** The acromial end of the clavicle is flat and the sternal end quadrangular in shape
- **b)** The weakest portion of the clavicle is the lateral third
- **c)** The coracoclavicular ligament supports the acromioclavicular joint
- **d)** Posterior dislocation of the sternoclavicular joint can cause injury to the great vessels of the superior mediastinum

30 With regards to X-rays of the lower limb
- **a)** A lipohaemarthrosis of the knee is only visible on the lateral X-ray
- **b)** It is important to distinguish between an intertrochanteric fracture and a subcapital fracture of the neck of femur
- **c)** Any talar shift seen on a fractured ankle is of significance
- **d)** A fracture of the base of the fifth metatarsal in a child can be differentiated from an epiphysis by its longitudinal position

31 The following describes the mechanism of excitation of specialised sensory receptors

a) Compression of the nerve fibre momentarily increases the permeability of the fibre membrane

b) Due to the increased permeability, sodium ions flow freely to the outside of the fibre

c) Sodium ion movement sets up a local current flow between the point of high fibre permeability and the first node of Ranvier further up the fibre

d) The current flow creates a voltage across the fibre membrane which in turn elicits a series of action potentials

32 The blood brain barrier

a) Is penetrated easily by dopamine

b) Breaks down in areas of infection

c) Can be temporarily disrupted by IV injection of hypertonic fluids

d) Is fully developed at birth

33 Regarding peripheral nerve injuries

a) Injury to the dorsal scapular nerve causes winging of the scapula

b) Foot drop is caused by injury to the common fibular nerve

c) The sciatic nerve is a branch of the lumbar plexus

d) The complete severing of spinal cord at C6 causes respiratory arrest

34 The following is true in schistosomiasis

a) Schistosomules mature into adult forms in the lungs

b) *S. haematobium* chronic infection can lead to obstructive uropathy

c) Praziquantel is the drug of choice

d) 'Swimmer's itch' is the first clinical sign

35 Regarding herpes viruses

a) Herpes simplex virus 1 can cause dendritic corneal ulcer

b) Postherpetic neuralgia is a complication of herpes zoster

c) The infective period in chicken pox is from onset of rash until all the lesions are at crusting stage

d) Cytomegalovirus is considered to cause oral hairy leukoplakia in AIDS patients

36 The internal jugular vein

a) Has the last four cranial nerves as medial relations at the base of the skull

b) Receives the anterior jugular vein

c) Is a continuation of the transverse cranial venous sinus

d) Lies medial to the styloid process and its muscles

37 Regarding the ear

a) The external auditory meatus is about 5 cm long

b) The outer 3/4 of the canal is cartilaginous

c) The tympanic membrane consists of three layers

d) One can visualise the underlying malleus and part of stapes using an auroscope

38 Regarding coagulation disorders

a) Antithrombin III is an inhibitor of activated factor X and thrombin

b) Myeloproliferative disorders predispose to both arterial and venous thrombosis

c) 'Lupus' anticoagulant in SLE predisposes to a bleeding tendency

d) Activation of platelet cyclo-oxygenase prevents platelet aggregation

39 Regarding complications of blood transfusion

a) Febrile reactions are usually due to antibodies to leucocytes or platelets

b) Blood group incompatibility can cause haemolytic destruction of donor cells or recipient cells

c) Transfusion haemosiderosis occurs in patients requiring repeated transfusion for blood loss

d) In mild allergic reactions transfusion can be continued slowly

40 As regards the pathophysiology of fracture healing

a) The fracture haematoma is vascularised by ingrowth of blood vessels from the surrounding tissues

b) Mobility at the fracture site causes subperiosteal new bone formation

c) The callus tends to be large in children

d) Remodelling of bone is better in adults than in children

41 The following are true about the basal metabolic rate (BMR)

a) The normal BMR at rest is 60–70 calories/min

b) Thyroid hormones cause the most significant change in BMR than all the other hormones excluding adrenaline and noradrenaline

c) The BMR can be elevated by up to 10 times normal with very high temperatures

d) Exercise is the most powerful stimulus for increasing BMR

42 The following is true in an electrocardiogram

a) Erythromycin prolongs QT interval

b) Normal QRS duration is up to 140 milliseconds

c) ST segment should not deviate by more than 1 mm above or below the isoelectric line in any lead

d) The normal PR interval is 120–200 milliseconds

43 The following are normal biochemistry values in serum

a) Potassium 3.0–5.0 mmol/L

b) Bilirubin 2–30 μmol/L

c) Sodium 135–145 mmol/L

d) Calcium 2.2–2.6 mmol/L

44 HIV testing

a) Should be offered in the emergency department

b) IgM antibodies are the basis of current blood tests

c) Antibodies may appear around 6 weeks after exposure

d) CD4 counts provide an indication of disease progression

45 The liver

a) The fossa of the gallbladder is covered with peritoneum

b) The quadrate lobe has the groove for the inferior vena cava to its right

c) The subphrenic and hepatorenal recesses do not communicate

d) The portal vein enters the liver at the porta hepatis

46 The sympathetic nervous system

a) Extends as a chain from the base of the skull to the coccyx

b) Has efferent fibres which are vasoconstrictor to skin arterioles, sudomotor to sweat glands and pilomotor to cutaneous hair

c) Has some preganglionic fibres which end in direct contact with the chromaffin adrenal medullary cells
d) Has its fibres interrupted as they pass to the eyelid and pupil in Horner's syndrome

47 In haemorrhagic shock
a) The resulting lactic acidosis decreases the peripheral vascular responsiveness to catecholamines
b) The arterial baroreceptors are stretched to a greater degree and sympathetic output is increased
c) Vasoconstriction is most marked in the gut
d) The initial decrease in urine output is due mostly to the haemodynamic alterations in the kidneys

48 Regarding renal functions
a) The glomerular filtration rate fluctuates throughout the day
b) Serum urea concentration is an excellent measure of glomerular function
c) Up to 200 mg of albumin may be found normally in a 24-hour urine specimen
d) Parathyroid hormone promotes tubular reabsorption of phosphate

49 Pharmacokinetics consider
a) The effect of the drug on the body and the mode of drug action
b) The proportion of administered drug that is available to have an effect
c) The ability of the body to eliminate the drug and its volume of distribution
d) The way in which the body affects a drug by the process of absorption, distribution, metabolism and excretion

50 Etomidate
a) Comes as a clear aqueous solution but is unstable in water
b) Depresses the synthesis of cortisol even after a single bolus dose
c) Can often cause moderate or severe involuntary movements on induction of anaesthesia
d) May be used safely in patients with porphyria

Practice Paper 3

1 Regarding leukaemias

a) The characteristic cell in chronic granulocytic leukaemia is the myelocyte

b) In acute leukaemia the onset of symptoms may be abrupt or insidious

c) In acute leukaemia the total white cell count at the onset can be subnormal

d) According to the FAB classification, on bone marrow examination, a proportion of blast cells of 50% or more is essential for the diagnosis of acute leukaemia

2 In myocardial infarction

a) The diagnostic sensitivity of troponins at 12 hours after onset of chest pain is 100%

b) The underlying mechanism is plaque rupture leading to thrombus formation

c) One of the ECG criteria for diagnosis is 1 mm ST elevation in two or more contiguous chest leads

d) Thrombolysis can be initiated up to 24 hours from onset of chest pain

3 Cyanosis can be seen in

a) Tetralogy of Fallot

b) Methaemoglobinaemia

c) Sulphaemoglobinaemia

d) Massive pulmonary embolism

4 In the skull

a) The falx cerebri and the tentorium cerebelli are formed by the meningeal layer of the duramater

b) The cranial venous sinuses eventually drain into the external jugular vein

c) The subarachnoid space is between the arachnoid and the dura

d) The arachnoid granulations drain the cerebrospinal fluid into the venous system

5 The sciatic nerve
a) Is posterior to the quadratus femoris muscle
b) Gives an articular branch to the hip joint
c) Crosses a point midway between the posterior superior iliac spine and the ischial tuberosity
d) Can be damaged by an IM injection to the upper outer quadrant of the buttock

6 The following contacts of patients of meningococcal meningitis require chemoprophylaxis
a) People in the same household
b) School, nursery or playgroup contacts
c) Kissing contacts
d) All health care staff involved in patient care

7 Regarding worm infections
a) Pruritus ani is usually the only symptom in whipworm infection
b) Mebendazole or pyrantel pamoate is used to treat whipworm infection
c) *Enterobius vermicularis* is transmitted by the faeco-oral route
d) *Trichuris trichiura* life-cycle passes through human lungs

8 The following is true of benzodiazepines
a) They all undergo biotransformation in the liver before excretion
b) Most are transformed to inactive metabolites
c) Midazolam and lorazepam are short-acting
d) Diazepam has an elimination half-life of 24 hours

9 Drug absorption after ingestion
a) Occurs predominantly in the colon
b) Peptides are well absorbed after oral administration
c) Is usually complete after 90 minutes
d) Is most commonly through passive diffusion

10 The following is true in respiratory pathophysiology
a) Physiological dead space = Anatomical dead space − Alveolar dead space
b) The amount of oxygen in solution in plasma is very low
c) The PaO_2 is the best indicator of alveolar ventilation

d) The normal alveolar arterial oxygen gradient increases with age

11 Regarding renal tubular functions

a) In diabetes insipidus, the urine:plasma osmolality ratio is more than 2

b) Aminoaciduria is seen in Fanconi syndrome

c) In type II renal tubular acidosis there is defective hydrogen ion secretion in the distal tubule

d) 50% of the glomerular filtrate is reabsorbed in the renal tubules

12 In patients with a fever

a) Antibiotics should always be given

b) It is important to reduce the body temperature as quickly as possible as to reduce the risk of seizure

c) A blood culture is more likely to be positive if it is done whilst the patient has a fever

d) Adults with suspected bacterial meningitis should have 10 mg IV dexamethasone prior to antibiotics to improve neurological outcome

13 Clinical features and signs in acute appendicitis

a) Cullen's sign is positive

b) Rovsing's sign can be positive

c) Can start with central abdominal pain

d) Psoas' test shows pain on hyperextension of left hip

14 Regarding formation of blood cells

a) The mature granulocytes are produced by proliferation and maturation of myeloblasts

b) The monocytes and macrophages are mainly distributed to the extravascular space

c) Mature plasma cells are derived from lymphoblasts

d) Decrease in the oxygen-carrying capacity of blood stimulates erythropoietin production

15 Regarding sickle-cell disease

a) In sickle-cell disease the oxygen dissociation curve is shifted to the right

b) In sickle-cell trait the sickle test and the haemoglobin solubility test are negative

c) Chronic haemolytic anaemia is seen in sickle-cell disease
d) Autosplenectomy occurs at a young age

16 In surface anatomy of the abdomen
a) The transpyloric plane passes through the L1 vertebra
b) The aorta bifurcates at the level of L3 vertebra
c) The deep inguinal ring lies superior to the inguinal ligament at the mid-inguinal point
d) The spleen follows the contour of the eighth rib on the left posterior to the mid-axillary line

17 In the forearm
a) The pronator teres is supplied by the ulnar nerve
b) The flexor pollicis longus originates from the anterior surface of the ulna
c) The anterior interosseous nerve innervates the pronator quadratus
d) Anconeus is situated in the deep layer of the posterior compartment

18 The femoral triangle
a) Has the medial border of iliopsoas as the lateral boundary
b) Contains the femoral nerve in its femoral sheath
c) Has the femoral canal as its most medial structure
d) Can have a femoral hernia which can be distinguished from an inguinal hernia because its neck is always medial to the pubic tubercle

19 Regarding validity of a study
a) Random error will reduce with increasing sample size
b) Bias will make *p* values and confidence intervals misleading
c) Confounding is reduced by true randomisation
d) Selection bias is a form of systematic error

20 Local factors that impede wound healing are
a) Decreased skin tension
b) Damage to the sensory nerves around the wound
c) Decreased local mobility
d) The presence of necrotic tissue

21 Adenosine
a) Is a purine nucleoside
b) Has a half-life of approximately 1 minute

c) When used with patients on dipyridamole need to have higher doses as it blocks adenosine receptors
d) Can be used to help slow atrial fibrillation

22 Metformin
a) May cause lactic acidosis
b) Does not stimulate insulin secretion
c) Is safe to be prescribed for patients with alcoholism
d) Inhibits hepatic gluconeogenesis

23 Regarding acid–base balance
a) Renal correction of either acidosis or alkalosis is dependent on a normal glomerular filtration rate
b) The renal tubular cell secretes H^+ ions into the urine in exchange for Na^+ ions
c) In erythrocytes, the H^+ ion produced by the carbonate dehydratase mechanism is buffered by haemoglobin
d) Normal urine is bicarbonate free

24 Regarding the spinal cord
a) The posterior columns comprise a medial and lateral tract called the fasciculus cuneatus and fasciculus gracilis respectively
b) The sensory fibres of the posterior columns decussate in the medulla
c) All the motor fibres decussate in the brain stem before descending in the cord
d) A penetrating injury here can cause a hemisection of the cord resulting in paralysis on the affected side below the lesion and loss of pain/temperature on the opposite side

25 Regarding dentition
a) All the deciduous teeth have appeared by 2 years
b) The first permanent tooth is the incisor or first molar at 8 years of age
c) The second permanent molar appears at 12 years of age
d) The periodontal membrane fixes each tooth in its socket and appears as a radiodense line seen around the root of each tooth on X-ray

26 The following is true about normal blood gas values
a) pH is 7.30 to 7.40
b) pCO_2 is 4.6 to 6.0 kPa

c) pO_2 is 9.0 to 12.5 kPa
d) Base excess is −2.0 to +2.0 mmol/L

27 Typical CSF changes in meningitis
a) Glucose is less than half of blood glucose in viral meningitis
b) CSF can appear clear in viral meningitis
c) Tuberculous meningitis has more polymorphs than mononuclear cells in CSF
d) In bacterial meningitis the CSF protein is <0.4 g/L

28 The following can present with abdominal pain
a) Herpes zoster
b) Myocardial infarction
c) Pleurisy
d) Superior mesenteric artery embolism

29 According to the immunisation schedule
a) Measles, mumps and rubella vaccine should be given around 13 months of age
b) The first dose of pneumococcal conjugate vaccine should be given at 2 months of age
c) Hepatitis B vaccine to be given at birth to babies whose mothers are at high risk of having hepatitis B
d) BCG vaccination at birth to all babies who are likely to come in contact with cases of TB

30 Syphilis
a) Has an incubation period of 4–8 weeks
b) Presents with a chancre on the genitalia or anus and causes regional tender and enlarged lymph nodes
c) In the secondary stage may present with any of the following: a maculopapular rash; condylomata lata; widespread lymphadenopathy and skin granulomas
d) Is caused by treponema pallidum and treated with penicillin

31 The rectum
a) Is related posteriorly to the third, fourth and fifth sacral nerves
b) Has a venous drainage into the superior mesenteric vein
c) Begins in front of the second sacral vertebra
d) Is covered anteriorly by peritoneum along its entire length

32 The left phrenic nerve
- **a)** Descends through the thorax in the left pleural cavity
- **b)** Receives sensory branches from the diaphragmatic peritoneum
- **c)** Passes through the caval opening of the diaphragm
- **d)** Arises from the dorsal rami of the third, fourth and fifth cervical nerves

33 Causes of eosinophilia include
- **a)** Malaria
- **b)** Hodgkin's disease
- **c)** Scabies
- **d)** Loeffler's syndrome

34 In haemolytic disease of the newborn
- **a)** The majority of cases are due to Rh incompatibility
- **b)** Haemolytic disease of the newborn due to ABO incompatibility commonly occurs with the first pregnancy
- **c)** The maternal IgM antibodies cross the placenta and react with foetal red cells
- **d)** Can occur due to anti-Kell and anti-S antibodies

35 According to the Salter–Harris classification of epiphyseal injuries
- **a)** Type 1 is crushing of part or all of the epiphysis
- **b)** Type 2 is the commonest injury
- **c)** Type 3 is a separation of part of the epiphyses
- **d)** Type 4 is one in which the whole epiphysis is separated from the shaft

36 Cyclic AMP performs the following intracellular function
- **a)** Activates enzymes
- **b)** Alters the permeability of cell membranes
- **c)** Activates protein synthesis
- **d)** Alters the degree of smooth muscle contraction

37 Regarding reflexes
- **a)** A muscle jerk can be elicited in any skeletal muscle by suddenly striking its tendon or the muscle itself
- **b)** The extensor thrust reflex helps support the body against gravity
- **c)** The crossed extensor reflex occurs when an extensor reflex occurs in one limb, impulses pass to the opposite side of the cord

and stimulate interneurons controlling the extensor muscles of the opposite limb

d) Tendon reflexes can be inhibited by the brain

38 The response to acute severe haemorrhage includes

a) The release of thromboxane A1, activating platelets and controlling bleeding vessels

b) Increased release of ADH from the anterior pituitary

c) The increase in renin secretion from the juxtaglomerular cells in the kidneys

d) An increase in base line vagal tone

39 Tetanus prone wounds are

a) Those less than 6 hours old

b) Puncture wound on the buttock

c) Those with devitalised tissue

d) Sustained in farms

40 The narrowest part of the male urethra is at

a) The internal urethral orifice

b) The navicular fossa

c) The site of the colliculus seminalis

d) The level of the perineal membrane

41 The cerebral hemispheres

a) Consists of four lobes

b) The frontal lobe has all cortical areas in front of the central sulcus of Rolando

c) The parietal lobe is mainly concerned with somatic sensation

d) Paraplegia may result from very midline lesions, like sagittal sinus thrombosis

42 The femoral artery

a) Is a continuation of the common iliac artery

b) Is located at the midpoint of the inguinal ligament

c) Gives off the profunda femoris branch which provides collateral circulation by anastomosing with the popliteal artery

d) Is often injured with fractures of the femoral shaft

43 Referred pain

a) Occurs when a visceral sensation is transmitted through a visceral pathway via sensory autonomic fibres to an area remote from the organ

b) From the heart is typically felt in the left shoulder and left arm because of its embryonic development in this area
c) Is visceral pain and one of the most important stimulus for this is ischaemia
d) Can be manifested as headache

44 Synovium
a) Lines joints, tendon sheaths and bursae
b) Secretes a viscous fluid rich in hyaluronan
c) Is not permeable to water
d) Has a net of small blood vessels beneath its surface cell layer

45 The following drugs can reduce glomerular filtration rate (GFR)
a) Ranitidine
b) Lisinopril
c) Iodine-containing contrast media
d) Naproxen

46 Suxamethonium
a) Is a non-depolarising neuromuscular blocking agent
b) Is broken down by plasma cholinesterase, an enzyme which is genetically controlled
c) Can cause complete skeletal muscle paralysis in 45 seconds
d) Causes a rise in potassium and intraocular pressures

47 Cardiac output is measured in man by
a) An electromagnetic flow meter placed over the ascending aorta
b) Using a Doppler and an echocardiogram
c) Injection of a dye and measuring its dilution over a period of time
d) Multiplying the oxygen consumption by the A–V difference of oxygen across the lungs

48 Causes of syncope include
a) Complete heart block with ventricular asystole
b) Pressure on the carotid sinus
c) Autonomic insufficiency
d) Increased stroke volume

49 The skin
a) Regulates the body temperature
b) Functions as an excretory organ

c) Is the most extensive and varied form of the sense organs
d) Produces vitamin D

50 About statistical tests
a) Pearson's coefficient of linear correlation is a non-parametric test
b) Chi-squared test is used to compare proportions or percentages between groups
c) Parametric tests usually assume that the data are normally distributed
d) Non-parametric tests are usually based on ranks

Practice Paper 4

1 HIV/AIDS

a) Progression to AIDS is defined by the development of two of the AIDS-defining illnesses

b) Only about 15% of AIDS patients develop *Pneumocystis carinii* pneumonia

c) Opportunistic infections are the most frequent complications of HIV infection

d) Diagnosis is based on detecting anti-HIV antibodies in the serum

2 Regarding acquired immunisation

a) BCG is a killed whole bacterial vaccine

b) The protective immunity conferred by the MMR vaccine lasts lifelong

c) Subunit vaccines are used for passive immunisation

d) Polio vaccine is made in both live and killed forms of the virus

3 Drugs that may interact with local anaesthetic agents are

a) Ketamine

b) Antiemetics

c) Calcium-channel blockers

d) Antihypertensive

4 Digoxin

a) Is a cardiac glycoside and inhibits sodium–potassium ATPase

b) Causes a reduction in intracellular calcium

c) Stimulates the vagus nerve and sensitises the baroreceptors

d) Takes up to 6 hours to achieve its peak effect if given orally but only 1 hour if given intravenously

5 In late diastole

a) The pressure in the ventricles are low

b) The mitral valve is shut

c) The aortic valve is closed
d) Blood stops filling the atria

6 Which of the following statements are true?
a) Patients taking calcium-channel blockers may not have a tachycardic response to haemorrhage
b) Elderly patients are less tolerant to hypovolaemia compared with the rest of the general population
c) Coagulopathies are common in the first hour of resuscitation in haemorrhagic shock
d) If a traumatic intra-abdominal injury is suspected a FAST (focused abdominal ultrasound examination) may be preferred in the unstable patient

7 Hypersecretion of adrenocortical hormones
a) Can result in primary hyperaldosteronism which causes hyponatraemia, hyperkalaemia, hypotension and a hyperdynamic circulation
b) Causes Cushing's disease resulting in hyperglycaemia, hypertension, weakness of tissues and loss of muscle bulk of the torso
c) Can cause adrenogenital syndrome if the adrenocortical cells form an androgen-secreting tumour
d) Results in cardiovascular collapse if the body undergoes severe stress

8 Regarding good medical practice
a) You must inform the GMC without delay if you have been charged with a criminal offence anywhere in the world
b) You are entitled to remain silent in an inquiry into a patient's death by the coroner or procurator fiscal when your evidence may lead to criminal proceedings being taken against you
c) When working in a team you must support colleagues who have problems with performance
d) You must treat information about patients as confidential even after their death

9 In anaemia
a) Koilonychia is most commonly seen in megaloblastic anaemia
b) Blood loss is the commonest cause of anaemia in clinical practice
c) The MCV and MCH are reduced in iron deficiency anaemia

d) Sideroblastic anaemia causes dimorphic red cell picture on peripheral blood film

10 Regarding the normal haemostatic mechanism

a) Platelet aggregation is dependent on the loss of the discoid platelet configuration and the formation of pseudopods

b) Glycoprotein IIb/IIIa complex is present in the platelet cytoplasm

c) Platelet adhesion is dependent on the von Willebrand factor

d) The damaged blood vessel undergoes a temporary reflex nervous vasodilatation

11 The following are true of the mandible

a) It has a vertical ramus which has an anterior coracoid and posterior condyloid process

b) It has a foramen on the medial aspect of the body for the inferior dental branch of the trigeminal nerve

c) It has a foramen on the lateral surface from which emerges the mental nerve

d) Osteomyelitis occurs only in the lower jaw after dental extractions of permanent teeth

12 Regarding the cerebral hemispheres

a) The auditory cortex lies in the posterior aspect of the frontal lobe

b) The hippocampal gyrus is the most medial part of the undersurface of the temporal lobe

c) Most areas of the cerebral cortex receive their main afferent input from the thalamus

d) Injury to the temporal lobes often results in patients being disinhibited

13 Regarding the foot

a) Inversion is mainly due to the action of tibialis anterior and tibialis posterior

b) Inversion and eversion occur at the talocalcaneal joint

c) The medial arch of the foot is supported by three tendons

d) Calcaneal fractures are typically caused by severe eversion of the foot

14 The validity of diagnostic studies is affected by

a) The selection of the 'gold' standard test

b) Spectrum of disease

c) Blinding of the assessors
d) Inclusion and exclusion criteria

15 Secondary closure of a wound
a) Is indicated when the skin edges are viable
b) After wound contraction has occurred gives a better cosmetic result
c) May be carried out for a healing abscess cavity
d) Can be done soon after debridement for gross contamination

16 Antagonists are drugs which
a) bind to the agonist to reduce its effect
b) bind to the same site as the agonist
c) have a greater affinity for the receptor than the agonist
d) bind to the receptor to reduce the actions of the agonist

17 Atropine is often required in the following poisonings
a) Organophosphate
b) Gamma-hydroxybutyric acid
c) Tricyclic antidepressant
d) Digoxin

18 Regarding heat loss from the body
a) By far the majority of heat loss is by radiation
b) The only means of maintaining normal body temperature when the environmental temperature is above body temperature is by evaporation of sweat
c) White clothing makes the body cooler than black clothing in hot weather
d) Wet clothes conduct heat away from the body twice as quickly as air

19 The pudendal canal
a) Can be injected with local anaesthetic to relieve the pain of childbirth
b) Is a space within the iliacus fascia
c) Is traversed by the nerve to the obturator internus
d) Lines the medial wall of the ischioanal fossa

20 The thoracic wall
a) Has a well-defined deep fascia
b) Transverse diameter is increased by the elevation of the vertebrosternal ribs (2–6)

c) Has five pairs of typical and seven pairs of atypical ribs
d) Has costochondral joints between each rib and its cartilage which are secondary cartilaginous joints

21 Regarding osmolality
a) The osmolality of the intracellular fluid is always the same as the extracellular fluid
b) The normal serum osmolality is about 250–260 milliosmoles/kg
c) In a 24-hour urine specimen the urine osmolality is usually higher than the serum osmolality
d) The osmolar gap is normally about 10 milliosmoles

22 Pulse oximetry
a) Uses a combination of plethysmography and spectrophotometry
b) Cannot distinguish between oxygenated haemoglobin, carboxyhaemoglobin and methaemoglobin
c) Is as accurate as invasive monitoring of oxygen
d) Is dependent on a pulsatile flow of blood

23 'Red flag' signs in a patient with back pain include
a) Thoracic pain
b) Ill health or presence of other medical illnesses
c) Disturbed gait
d) Age of onset between 20 and 55 years

24 The following is true in hepatitis A
a) It is most infectious just before the onset of jaundice
b) It is a notifiable disease
c) It progresses to chronic liver disease in about 1% of patients
d) The virus is killed by boiling water for 10 minutes

25 In meningitis
a) The glucose content of CSF is reduced in bacterial infections
b) A lumbar puncture should always be performed
c) Leptospirosis, typhus and amoeba can be the causative agents
d) Caused by meningococcus, the administration of intravenous dexamethasone before antibiotics reduces mortality

26 The elbow joint
a) The radial head is the first secondary ossification centre to appear at the age of about one year

b) The proximal radioulnar joint which is a part of the elbow joint is involved with pronation and supination of the forearm
c) Fat pads are located in the coronoid, olecranon and the radial fossae
d) The biceps brachii muscle acts as a powerful supinator of the forearm

27 The appendix
a) Is suspended from the caecum by the mesoappendix which contains the appendicular vessels
b) Is derived from the hindgut
c) Its position in relation to the caecum is variable
d) Has normally got large aggregations of lymphoid tissue

28 Regarding blood groups
a) ABO antigens are present on lymphocytes
b) Antigens C, D and E are Rhesus antigens
c) Anti-A and anti-B immune antibodies can be found after immunisation with tetanus toxoid
d) A1 and A2 are subgroups of blood group A

29 Regarding formation of blood cells
a) Androgens stimulate erythropoietin production
b) Newly formed blood cells enter circulation in the vascular sinusoids of the bone marrow
c) The skull and bones of the thorax predominantly contain red marrow
d) Prolonged inhalation of oxygen at high concentrations stimulates erythropoiesis

30 Regarding hypersensitivity reactions
a) Anaphylactic reaction is mediated by IgE antibodies
b) Transfusion reactions are an example of type II hypersensitivity
c) Acute serum sickness is caused by immune complex-mediated type III hypersensitivity
d) Type IV hypersensitivity is mediated by $CD4^+$ T-helper-1 cells

31 Growth hormone
a) Is secreted by the anterior pituitary and increases the size and number of all cells
b) Decreases the rate of carbohydrate utilisation by cells

c) Increases protein breakdown so there is a high turnover of cells during growth
d) Is controlled by the hypothalamus due to its secretion of growth hormone stimulating hormone

32 Respiratory acidosis
a) May be acute or chronic
b) Renal compensation takes 4–6 hours for full effect
c) Can be caused by choking
d) The PCO_2 may be normal or raised

33 The Frank–Starling curves
a) Show the relationship between systolic pressure and stroke volume
b) Are shifted downwards when contractility of the myocardium is increased
c) Cannot be applied to the transplanted heart
d) Are shifted to the left when digitalis is used

34 Rabies
a) Has an average incubation period of 1–3 months
b) Post-exposure prophylaxis is given as five doses of HDCV (1 mL) on day 0 and day 3, 7, 14 and 28 by IM injection
c) Is characterised by pain and tingling at the initial wound site in the prodromal period
d) Aerophobia (fear of air) is a pathognomonic feature

35 Concerning the middle ear
a) It is also known as the tympanic cavity
b) The three ossicles articulate with each other in the following order: malleus, incus and stapes – going externally to internally
c) The roof is formed by a thin sheet of bone separating it from the anterior cranial fossa
d) The Eustachian tube connects it to the nasopharynx and at this point there is considerable lymphoid tissue

36 Regarding the cervical vertebrae
a) They all have foramen transversarium through which passes the vertebral artery
b) With the exception of C1, they all have bifid spinous processes
c) Lateral flexion of the neck occurs at the atlantoaxial joint

d) Dislocation may occur without fracture because of the horizontal intervertebral facet joints

37 Pain

a) Can be perceived by all of the following stimuli: trauma to tissues, ischaemia, intense heat or cold and chemical irritation

b) Is perceived at different degrees of tissue damage by different people

c) Causes different reactivity in individuals

d) Pricking pain is perceived as different to burning pain because the former travels along fibres that pass through the reticular substance of the brainstem and the later terminates in the vertebrobasal complex of the thalamus

38 Cerebrospinal fluid

a) Is produced in the floor of the ventricles by the choroid plexus

b) Travels from the lateral ventricles through the third ventricle, the aqueduct of Sylvius and into the fourth ventricle

c) Is reabsorbed into the venous circulation through the arachnoid granulations that project into the cavernous sinus

d) Can have impaired reabsorption which can result in hydrocephalus

39 Lithium

a) Works by inhibiting the sodium–potassium pump mechanism

b) Is rapidly absorbed and excreted fully in the urine

c) Can cause neurogenic diabetes insipidus

d) Reduces the amplitude of T waves on ECG monitoring

40 Protamine

a) Is positively charged at physiological pH

b) Is used clinically to counteract the effects of heparin

c) Its interaction with heparin demonstrates chemical agonistic properties

d) Binds to a receptor in blood clots to prevent heparin from occupying it

41 In acute renal failure

a) Oliguria is defined as urine output less than 200 mL/day

b) In pre-renal failure the rise in urea is proportionally more than creatinine

c) Acute tubular necrosis causes severe hypokalaemia

d) Serum urea and creatinine levels may be initially normal in acute renal failure

42 Lung volumes and lung function tests

a) The vital capacity is the sum of inspiratory reserve volume and the tidal volume
b) The residual volume is measured with the help of a spirometer
c) FEV1/FVC ratio increases in obstructive airways disease
d) The tidal volume is usually about 6–8 mL/kg at rest

43 In the eyes

a) The cornea covers the anterior one-sixth of the surface of the eyeball
b) The superior oblique muscle medially rotates the eyeball
c) The aqueous humour is secreted in the anterior chamber and flows into the posterior chamber through the pupil
d) The macula lutea is the thinnest area of the retina with more rods than cones

44 Regarding the skin and its appendages

a) The nail grows from both the root and the proximal end of the nail bed
b) Spasm of the arrectores pilorum muscle produces 'goose skin'
c) The sebaceous glands are distributed mainly in the palms and soles
d) The ceruminous glands are modified sweat glands

45 Regarding statistics

a) The power of a study is the probability of correctly accepting the null hypothesis when it is false
b) Type I error is wrongly rejecting the null hypothesis
c) Type II error is wrongly accepting the null hypothesis
d) The *p* value is the probability of chance alone causing the observed effects in a trial

46 Causes of disseminated intravascular coagulation include

a) Heatstroke
b) Snake bite
c) Pulmonary embolism
d) Foetal death in utero

47 Causes of lymph node enlargement include

a) Sarcoidosis
b) Cat-scratch fever

c) Cytomegalovirus
d) Toxoplasmosis

48 The following are true in fundoscopy
a) Spontaneous retinal artery pulsations are frequently seen in normal eyes
b) Optic disc swelling is seen both in optic neuritis and papilloedema
c) Capillary microaneurysms are a characteristic feature of hypertensive retinopathy
d) In central retinal artery occlusion there is intense swelling of the optic disc

49 The anterior tibial artery
a) Is the larger of the two divisions of the popliteal artery
b) Becomes superficial just above the ankle joint lying between extensor hallucis longus and extensor digitorum
c) Continues on the dorsum of the foot as the dorsalis pedis pulse
d) Is commonly injured with direct blows to the anterior aspect of the lower leg

50 The pituitary gland
a) Has a large posterior and smaller anterior lobe
b) Has its two lobes connected by the pars infundibulum
c) Has the cavernous sinus laterally and the body of the petrous bone below
d) Can develop tumours which can compress the optic chiasma and cause poor visual acuity

Practice Paper 5

1 The following are true of urinary tract infections
  a) Most women with a UTI will also have vaginitis
  b) A negative leucocyte esterase on urine dipstick excludes the disease
  c) Nitrites on urine dipstick occur because of urease-splitting organisms such as proteus
  d) Pregnant patients should always be treated for bacteriuria even if asymptomatic

2 Pyrexia of unknown origin (PUO)
  a) In 25%, in some series, a diagnosis is not reached
  b) Drugs may be the cause of an increased temperature
  c) Is defined as a prolonged fever for over 2 weeks
  d) A subphrenic abscess is an unlikely cause

3 The common iliac arteries
  a) Give branches to the uterus in the female
  b) Are crossed at their origin by the ureters
  c) Arise in front of the sacral promontory
  d) Lie behind the internal iliac veins

4 With regards to the soft tissue structures of the vertebral column
  a) The peripheral part of the intervertebral disc is called annulus pulposus
  b) The ligamentum flavum links the spinous processes together
  c) Each articular facet is contained within small synovial joints
  d) A prolapsed intervertebral disc at L4/5 may cause numbness over the lateral part of the lower leg and medial aspect of the foot

5 In anaemias
  a) Tropical sprue causes megaloblastic anaemia
  b) Alcohol can cause macrocytosis by direct toxic effect on erythroblasts in the absence of folate deficiency

c) In rheumatoid arthritis the most common type of anaemia is microcytic hypochromic
d) Depression of erythropoiesis is the most important factor in anaemia of chronic renal failure

6 The following disorders cause paraproteinaemias
a) Primary amyloidosis
b) Benign monoclonal gammopathy
c) Multiple myeloma
d) Non-Hodgkin's lymphoma

7 About inflammatory markers
a) Low or normal levels of C-reactive protein rules out inflammation or infection
b) C-reactive protein is elevated by oral contraceptive pills
c) The amount of fibrinogen in the blood directly correlates with the ESR
d) The ESR is important in the diagnosis of temporal arteritis and polymyalgia rheumatica

8 With body temperature
a) Rectal temperature is generally 1°C above oral temperature
b) The anterior part of the hypothalamus is responsible for 'heat promotion' and mediates this through the sympathetic nervous system
c) All of the following occur to immediately increase body temperature: vasoconstriction of the skin vessels; sympathetic stimulation of the basal metabolic rate; shivering; piloerection and increased thyroid hormone production
d) When excessively hot the body can produce 1.5 L of sweat in a day

9 Regarding sodium homeostasis
a) Hypernatraemia can be caused by simultaneous loss of water and sodium
b) 8.4% sodium bicarbonate contains 1000 mmol/L of sodium
c) Primary hyperaldosteronism causes hyponatraemia
d) Urine osmolality is always very high in hypernatraemic patients

10 Regarding oxygen transport
a) 5% of oxygen in the blood is carried in the dissolved state
b) Fever reduces the affinity of haemoglobin to oxygen

- **c)** Increase in 2,3 DPG shifts the oxyhaemoglobin dissociation curve to the right
- **d)** Metabolic alkalosis reduces the affinity of haemoglobin to oxygen

11 Chlamydial infection

- **a)** Causes an increased risk of cervical cancer in women
- **b)** May present as right upper quadrant pain in men due to perihepatitis and called Fitz-Hugh and Curtis syndrome
- **c)** Is confirmed by cell culture and has a high sensitivity and rarely has false-negative results
- **d)** Should be treated with azithromycin or doxycycline

12 Regarding the scalp

- **a)** The auriculotemporal nerve supplies the scalp posterior to the ear
- **b)** The aponeurotic layer includes the occipitofrontalis muscle
- **c)** The superficial temporal artery supplying the scalp is a branch of the external carotid artery
- **d)** Bleeding from scalp lacerations is usually self-limiting

13 The posterior mediastinum

- **a)** Is continuous through the superior mediastinum with the neck
- **b)** Is traversed by the deep cardiac plexus of nerves
- **c)** Can be involved in neck infections spreading between the pretracheal and prevertebral fasciae
- **d)** Extends posteriorly down to T10 vertebra level

14 Cerebrospinal fluid

- **a)** Has more protein compared with plasma
- **b)** Raised intracranial pressure is a contraindication for performing a lumbar puncture
- **c)** Normal glucose level is >60% of blood level
- **d)** Shows predominantly lymphocytes in viral meningitis

15 Biomechanics

- **a)** Is concerned with the internal and external forces acting on the body
- **b)** When abnormal can lead to chronic injuries
- **c)** Should be considered in patellofemoral syndrome
- **d)** Also, deals with work energy and power

16 Ketamine

a) Is a phencyclidine derivative and binds to GABA receptors

b) Provides substantial analgesia and can be administered intramuscularly

c) Increases arterial pressure by 25% but reduces intracranial pressure

d) Can cause nightmares especially in children

17 Anticholinergic inhaled agents

a) Work by inhibiting the bronchoconstriction caused by stimulation of the vagus nerve

b) Reduce secretion of mucus

c) Ipratropium bromide is a derivative of atropine

d) Inhibit the rise in intracellular cyclic AMP

18 The cardiac output is determined by

a) Blood volume

b) Blood flow to cardiac muscle

c) Stroke volume

d) Heart rate

19 Which of the following occur in haemorrhagic shock?

a) Increased entry of blood into the circulating blood

b) Decreased secretion of glucagon

c) Decreased secretion of noradrenalin

d) Increased secretion of vasopressin

20 The diaphragm

a) Is innervated primarily by the phrenic nerve from the C1 to C3 spinal cord levels

b) The aorta passes posterior to the median arcuate ligament at the level of T12 vertebra

c) The inferior vena cava passes through a large opening at the level of T10 vertebra

d) Muscular components originate from the medial and lateral arcuate ligaments

21 The Carpal tunnel

a) Is formed by the flexor retinaculum and the distal ends of radius and ulna

b) The flexor pollicis longus tendon and the median nerve pass through the carpal tunnel

c) The ulnar nerve passes anterior to the flexor retinaculum
d) The median nerve is posterior to the tendons in the carpal tunnel

22 The validity of therapy studies is affected by
a) Randomisation
b) Duration of follow-up
c) Intention to treat
d) Blinding

23 Henoch–Schonlein syndrome
a) Females are affected more frequently than males
b) Purpura may be absent
c) Biopsy from involved kidney and skin shows IgG deposition
d) Is a self-limiting illness with no recurrence

24 In hyperthyroidism
a) If prolonged, it can cause a degenerative process to occur particularly of the myocardium
b) Exophthalmos occurs and resolves with treatment
c) Atrial fibrillation occurs but readily responds to cardioversion
d) Is most commonly caused by a thyroid adenoma

25 Causes of ulceration of throat include
a) Agranulocytic angina
b) Vincent's angina
c) Infectious mononucleosis
d) Diphtheria

26 The atlas vertebra
a) Has the first cervical spinal nerve posterior to the atlanto-occipital joint
b) Has the vertebral artery lying on its anterior arch
c) Has the alar ligament attached to it
d) Moves with the occipital bone on rotation of the head

27 Avulsion fractures of the pelvis occur
a) As a result of chronic stress in young athletes
b) At the anterior superior iliac spine
c) As a result of direct trauma
d) At the ischial tuberosity due to adductor brevis contracting severely

28 The following is true in needlestick injuries
- **a)** The risk of blood-borne virus transmission will reduce with exposure of the needle to sunlight
- **b)** Testing of the needle for the presence of blood-borne viruses is highly recommended
- **c)** Approximate risk of transmission of HIV from a known infected source and fresh blood on the needle is 3 per 1000
- **d)** Informed consent is mandatory before testing source patient for HIV

29 Regarding tapeworm infections
- **a)** Cerebral cysticercosis is caused by *T. saginata*
- **b)** *T. solium* inhabits the human upper jejunum
- **c)** Diphyllobothrium latum causes hydatid cysts in liver
- **d)** Niclosamide is used to treat *Taenia solium*

30 Regarding penicillins
- **a)** They mainly act by inhibiting cell wall synthesis
- **b)** They are very lipid-soluble
- **c)** They are rapidly excreted by the kidney
- **d)** Patients who are allergic to penicillin may not necessarily be allergic to cephalosporins because they have very slightly different β-lactam rings

31 Agents that induce drug metabolising enzymes are
- **a)** Phenytoin
- **b)** Corticosteroids
- **c)** Acute intake of alcohol
- **d)** Allopurinol

32 Control of breathing
- **a)** The respiratory centre is situated in the midbrain
- **b)** The central chemoreceptors respond to changes in blood carbon dioxide content
- **c)** Chyne-Stokes breathing can be seen in congestive heart failure
- **d)** The pneumotaxic centre has an excitatory effect on inspiration

33 Regarding deafness
- **a)** Conduction deafness can occur following recurrent blockages of the Eustachian tube which connects the middle ear with the nasopharynx

b) In the elderly nerve deafness occurs and this is especially for low frequency sounds
c) Conduction and nerve deafness can be differentiated easily using a tuning fork and one such test is Rinne's test
d) An audiometer emits sounds of different frequencies and can be used to calculate the hearing loss for each frequency

34 Regarding fundoscopy
a) The physiological cup occupies only the centre and is usually not greater than 60% of the disc size
b) Pseudo-swelling of the optic disc is seen in marked hypermetropia
c) Arteriovenous nipping in seen in proliferative diabetic retinopathy
d) Optic atrophy is seen in retinitis pigmentosa

35 The following tests can be used to test the integrity of the anterior cruciate ligament of the knee
a) Anterior drawer test
b) Lachman test
c) Pivot shift test
d) McMurray test

36 Regarding the red blood cell
a) Deficiency of glucose 6 phosphate dehydrogenase can cause haemolysis due to oxidant damage
b) A fall in pH increases the affinity of oxyhaemoglobin for oxygen
c) Glucose binds covalently with haemoglobin to form glycosylated haemoglobin
d) Echinocytes are red blood cells with spiny protrusions of membrane due to metabolic stresses

37 Causes of thrombocytopaenia include
a) Alcoholism
b) Massive blood transfusion
c) Multiple myeloma
d) Aplastic anaemia

38 The sciatic nerve
a) Is the largest peripheral nerve in the body
b) Passes through the greater sciatic foramen and under gluteus maximus

c) Divides into the tibial and lateral fibular nerves
d) May be injured by posterior dislocation of the hip

39 The popliteal fossa
a) Has the tendons of semi-membranosus and semi-tendinosus as its supero-lateral border
b) Has its fascial roof pierced by the short saphenous vein
c) Has the common peroneal nerve passing out of the fossa along the biceps tendon
d) Contains a nerve, artery, vein in that order going from superficial to deep

40 The external carotid artery
a) Is crossed superficially by the hypoglossal nerve
b) Has the stylopharyngeus muscle passing between it and the internal carotid artery
c) Terminates by dividing into superficial temporal and transverse facial arteries
d) Lies lateral to the retromandibular vein

41 The following is true in research methods
a) Randomisation means random sampling
b) Sample attrition refers to loss of sample members before the post-test phase
c) Postal questionnaire eliminates interviewer bias
d) The dependant variable is also known as the intervention

42 Regarding T lymphocytes
a) Arise in the thymus and then migrate to bone marrow for maturation
b) T cells produce five different classes of immunoglobulins
c) Cytokines released by Helper T cells activate B cells and macrophages
d) The paracortex of a lymph node has abundance of T lymphocytes

43 Regarding antipsychotic agents
a) Almost all work by stimulating post-synaptic dopamine receptors
b) Chlorpromazine has four metabolites
c) Most have unwanted side effects which include cycloplegia, dry mouth, difficulty with micturition and impotence
d) They can be used to aid withdrawal from alcohol and other drugs

44 Insulin

a) Increases circulating free fatty acids
b) Causes glycogenolysis in the liver
c) Is released from pancreatic B cells at a low basal rate
d) Is a polypeptide hormone arranged in two chains linked by disulphide bridges

45 The stress response of the body to pain, injury or disease involves

a) Stimulation of the hypothalamus to secrete ACTH which in turn stimulates the adrenal cortex to secrete cortisol
b) Secretion of glucocorticoids to mobilise glucose and increase its utilisation by tissues
c) Stabilisation of lysosomal membranes by cortisol to prevent release of digestive enzymes which will autolyse internal structures of the cell
d) Adrenocortical stimulation which increases the availability of amino acids and fats to help repair tissues

46 Surface markings on chest examination include

a) The suprasternal notch is at the level of T2 vertebrae
b) The level of both aortic arch and bifurcation of the trachea are at T4 vertebrae
c) The manubriosternal joint is at the level of T3 vertebrae
d) During respiration the bifurcation moves between T4 and T6 vertebrae levels

47 The cerebellum

a) Surface is divided into numerous narrow folds called rugae
b) Is made up of two cerebellar hemispheres joined to each other
c) Is connected to the brainstem by three pairs of cerebral peduncles with the middle pair connecting it to the midbrain
d) Receives all its blood supply from the basilar artery

48 Regarding the pupil of the eye

a) Constriction of the pupil is caused by contraction of the radial muscle fibres
b) Some optic nerve impulses go directly to the pretectal nuclei in the brainstem
c) The iris can only constrict until the pupillary diameter is 3 mm
d) The pupillary light reflex is often absent in patients with syphilis of the central nervous system because of its predilection for destroying the oculomotor nerve fibres

49 The end-diastolic volume is increased by

a) Standing

b) Increasing intrapericardial pressure

c) Increased total blood volume

d) Decreased ventricular compliance

50 Regarding clinical symptoms and signs

a) Familial Mediterranean fever may present with pleuritic chest pain

b) Anisocoria is always pathological

c) Trousseau's sign is an indication of latent tetany

d) Clubbing of fingers is found in all cases of infective endocarditis

Practice Paper 6

1 Systemic factors that delay wound healing are
- **a)** Obesity
- **b)** Vitamin B deficiency
- **c)** Anticoagulants
- **d)** Rheumatoid arthritis

2 Propofol
- **a)** Is a phenol derivative and is an aqueous emulsion containing soya bean
- **b)** Causes a delay in the disappearance of the eyelash reflex
- **c)** Can cause significant hypotension due to marked myocardial depression
- **d)** Induces unconsciousness rapidly and its effects wear off quickly due to redistribution to other tissues

3 Drug antagonism
- **a)** Can occur with pharmacokinetic interference
- **b)** May be potentially irreversible
- **c)** Can occur with chemical antagonism
- **d)** Can occur as a result of interaction with receptor sites

4 Regarding fever
- **a)** It can be caused by infection, pulmonary embolism and after a myocardial infarction
- **b)** It occurs because substances such as polysaccharides or abnormal proteins reset the hypothalamic thermostat to a higher temperature level
- **c)** Rigors occur because the body tries to elevate the temperature even further to destroy the infectious agents
- **d)** Skin vasodilatation and sweating occur to try and combat the fever

5 Regarding the surface anatomy in the neck
- **a)** The inferior margin of the mandible forms the base of each anterior triangle

b) The cricothyroid membrane is located just superior to the thyroid notch
c) The jugular venous pulse is measured in the external jugular vein
d) The thyroid and parathyroid glands are present in the muscular triangle of the neck

6 Regarding the arterial tree in the abdomen
a) The lumbar arteries arise from the internal iliac arteries
b) The testicular artery is a branch of the renal artery
c) The common hepatic artery is a branch of the celiac trunk
d) The aorta bifurcates into the internal iliac arteries at the level of L4 vertebra

7 Regarding potassium homeostasis
a) Metabolic acidosis causes hyperkalaemia
b) Addison's disease causes hypokalaemia
c) Both hyperkalaemia and hypokalaemia cause muscle weakness
d) In hyperkalaemia, infusion of calcium gluconate reduces the potassium concentration

8 Type I respiratory failure
a) PaO_2 <8 kPa and $PaCO_2$ > 6.7 kPa
b) Is seen in early stages of severe asthma
c) Can be caused by ventilation/perfusion mismatch
d) Is treated by increasing the FiO_2

9 In a child with a fever
a) Ideally, both paracetamol and ibuprofen should be given together to reduce the temperature as they act synergistically
b) For suspected meningococcal septicaemia, cefotaxime is the preferred antibiotic
c) It is important to get blood cultures as soon as possible
d) For a suspected urinary tract infection, the urine should be obtained using urine bags

10 Investigations for suspected TB include
a) Biopsies of solid lesions and lymph nodes
b) Gastric washings subjected to staining and culture
c) Chest X-ray
d) Sputum culture in Ziehl–Nielsen medium

11 Osteomyelitis
- **a)** Is never caused by fungi, viruses and other parasites
- **b)** Is an infection of the cortex of a bone
- **c)** Is common in children due to haemophilus
- **d)** May originate from a small lesion such as a boil on the skin

12 At the shoulder joint
- **a)** The deltoid muscle initiates abduction
- **b)** The subacromial bursa does not communicate with the articular cavity
- **c)** The teres minor and teres major muscles form a part of the rotator cuff
- **d)** Anterior dislocations may lead to a radial nerve palsy

13 The autonomic nervous system
- **a)** Differs from the cerebrospinal nervous system by having the course of its efferent nerves interrupted by a synapse in a peripheral ganglion
- **b)** Has its sympathetic motor cells in the anterior grey columns of all the thoracic and upper two lumbar segments
- **c)** Has its cranial parasympathetic outflow along cranial nerves III, VIII, IX and X
- **d)** All sympathetic postganglionic terminals release adrenaline and noradrenaline

14 About chronic granulocytic leukaemia
- **a)** The platelet count can be normal to high
- **b)** Philadelphia chromosome is present in the neoplastic cells
- **c)** Blast crisis is more common in chronic lymphocytic leukaemia
- **d)** Splenomegaly is common

15 Causes of polycythaemia include
- **a)** Non-neoplastic kidney disease
- **b)** Chronic pulmonary disease
- **c)** High altitude
- **d)** Benign familial polycythaemia

16 Regarding immunodeficiencies
- **a)** In DiGeorge's syndrome, B cells and immunoglobulin levels are usually normal
- **b)** Wiskott–Aldrich syndrome is characterised by thrombocytopenia, eczema and recurrent infections

c) X-linked agammaglobulinaemia starts presenting at 8–9 months of age
d) $CD8^+$ helper T-cell depletion is central to the pathogenesis of AIDS

17 Cortisol
a) Increases the quantity of protein in most tissues in the body
b) Has its main function to increase resistance of the body to any physical stress
c) Depresses utilisation of glucose by tissues
d) Stabilises lysosomal membranes

18 With somaesthetic sensation there are several specialised tactile receptors
a) The pacinian corpuscle is quite superficial in tissues and responds to rapid tissue deformation
b) The meissner corpuscle is found in the toes and enables us to discriminate very precise texture and fine details of objects touched
c) Krause's corpuscles are located in the sexual organs and are responsible for some sexual sensations
d) Ruffini's end-organ detects stretch of tissues and joints allowing determination of the degree of angulation of the joint

19 Refractory shock
a) Can occur only with haemorrhagic shock
b) Causes damage to the gastrointestinal mucosa allowing bacteria to enter the circulation
c) Is a state when there is no longer any response to vasopressors despite correcting the blood volume
d) Is contributed to by negative feedback mechanisms of the CNS

20 Regarding infections with *Salmonella*
a) *S. typhimurium* causes acute gastroenteritis
b) Humans are the only known reservoirs of *S. typhi*
c) Chronic carriers are individuals who excrete *Salmonella* for at least 6 months
d) Fever with relative bradycardia is seen in patients with typhoid

21 The femoral nerve
a) Arises from the posterior divisions of L2, L3 and L4
b) Breaks up into its branches before it enters the femoral triangle

- **c)** Supplies only two of the three vasti muscles of the thigh
- **d)** Supplies the skin over the patella via the patella plexus

22 The temporomandibular joint

- **a)** Has a fibrocartilaginous articular disc dividing the joint into medial and lateral compartments
- **b)** Allows for movement from side-to-side as well as protrusion and retraction of the mandible
- **c)** Is easily visualised on an orthopantomogram
- **d)** When dislocated bilaterally presents with inability to open the mouth

23 The rennin–angiotensin–aldosterone system regulates

- **a)** Sodium balance
- **b)** Blood pressure
- **c)** Potassium balance
- **d)** Nitrogen balance

24 Equilibrium formation

- **a)** Is an essential function of the bulboreticular formation
- **b)** Is helped by the utricle and saccule which house special sensory structures called the crista ampullaris
- **c)** Is also helped by the three semicircular canals and particularly apprises the CNS of sudden changes in direction
- **d)** These sensory structures (utricle, saccule and semicircular canals) also convey information directly to the cerebellum and specifically helps the CNS to correct imbalance when it happens

25 Antipsychotic drugs can have drug interactions such as

- **a)** Respiratory depression if used with antihistamines or alcohol
- **b)** Increased anticholinergic effects with lithium
- **c)** Worsened orthostatic hypotension with tricyclic antidepressants
- **d)** Thioridazine and quinidine may cause hypokalaemia

26 Regarding inhaled bronchodilators

- **a)** The optimal size of particles used in aerosol bronchodilator therapies is 10–20 μm
- **b)** 50% of the total dose of aerosol particles are deposited in the mouth and pharynx
- **c)** Terbutaline is a β2 agonist and can be administered subcutaneously

d) β2 agonists inhibit the release of broncho-constricting substances from mast cells

27 In complete heart block

a) The conduction block can be at the level of the bundle of His
b) The ventricular rate is slower than the atrial rate
c) Fainting may occur due to prolonged periods during which the ventricles fail to contract
d) Fainting may occur because the atria are unable to pump blood into the ventricles

28 The following may be seen on an ECG in the normal healthy individual

a) Sinoatrial exit block
b) Mobitz type 1 AV block
c) Right bundle branch block
d) Right axis deviation

29 Ureters

a) Are constricted as they cross the common iliac vessels at the pelvic brim
b) The visceral afferent fibres return from T9 to T10 spinal cord levels
c) 90% of calculi are radio-opaque
d) Originate from the renal pelvis which lies anterior to the renal vessels

30 The subclavian vein

a) Receives the cephalic vein
b) Forms the brachiocephalic vein at the level of the first intercostal space
c) Is crossed anteriorly by the phrenic nerve
d) Receives the external jugular vein

31 In distribution of data

a) The mean is a good measure of central tendency in skewed distributions
b) The mean is higher than the median in negatively skewed distributions
c) Many distributions have more than one mode
d) The mean is the arithmetic average of all the numeric data

32 In diagnosing coagulation disorders
- **a)** Prothrombin time is prolonged in deficiency of factors VIII and IX
- **b)** Prolonged activated partial thromboplastin time with normal prothrombin time is suggestive of deficiency of factors II and V
- **c)** Thrombin time helps to determine levels of thrombin in the blood
- **d)** Specific coagulation factor assays are necessary to identify the deficient coagulation factor and the degree of deficiency

33 Regarding ENT conditions
- **a)** In quinsy the uvula is pulled to the affected side
- **b)** Epistaxis commonly starts at Little's area of the anterior inferior septum containing Kiesselbach's plexus
- **c)** Acute laryngotracheobronchitis is most commonly seen in the 11- to 16-year age group
- **d)** Autophony is a sensation of sound in the absence of an appropriate auditory stimulus

34 The following is true regarding brain stem death
- **a)** Heart continues to beat and spontaneous respirations are present
- **b)** No pupillary response to light
- **c)** No gag reflex
- **d)** No vestibulo-ocular response

35 The lymph drainage of the head and neck
- **a)** The right jugular duct opens directly into the jugular or subclavian vein
- **b)** The nodes are arranged from the sub-mental group to the occipital group
- **c)** The deep chain of lymph nodes is situated around the internal jugular vein
- **d)** Includes a circular chain of lymph nodes around the nasopharynx

36 With regards to the joints of the thorax
- **a)** The 12th costotransverse joint is a fibrocartilaginous joint
- **b)** The manubriosternal joint is a synovial joint
- **c)** The costovertebral joints are supplied by ventral rami
- **d)** The costochondral joints are synovial joints

37 Regarding infections in the immunocompromised patients
- **a)** The predominant pathogens in immunocompromised patients vary by the type of immunosuppression

b) Broad-spectrum antibiotic use decreases the risk of secondary fungal infections
c) Fever is often the only symptom of infection in the immunocompromised patient
d) Severe neutropenia is defined as an absolute neutrophil count below $1000/mm^3$

38 The following is true in pulmonary infections
a) Most lobar pneumonias are caused by pneumococci
b) One of the stages in the natural history of lobar pneumonia is red hepatisation
c) Lung abscesses can cause secondary amyloidosis
d) Cryptogenic organising pneumonia is caused by the fungus Cryptococcus

39 Aspirin overdose may cause
a) Coma
b) Pulmonary oedema
c) Jaundice
d) Thrombocytopaenia

40 Corticosteroids inhibit
a) Neutrophil production
b) Histamine release
c) Leukotrine C4 and D4 synthesis
d) Platelet thromboxane A2 synthesis

41 The following is true of the basal ganglia
a) The caudate nucleus controls fine intentional movements of the body
b) The putamen operates independently of the caudate nucleus
c) The globus pallidus controls the 'background' positioning of the body when a person begins to perform a complex movement
d) The subthalamic nucleus controls some aspects of speech

42 Regarding abnormalities in vision
a) Myopia is usually caused by an eyeball that is too long
b) Astigmatism occurs when the lens becomes ovoid in shape and the eye cannot focus clearly on an object regardless of how far away it is
c) Hypermetropia occurs when the lens bends the light rays too much
d) A concave lens is used to correct hypermetropia

43 The following are symptoms and signs of hyperthyroidism
- **a)** Intolerance to cold
- **b)** Lid lag
- **c)** Weight gain
- **d)** Tachycardia

44 The following is true in common presenting complaints
- **a)** Angina at rest is classed as Class 3 by the New York Heart Association
- **b)** Todd's paresis may persist for up to 24 hours
- **c)** Hypoglycaemia can be the cause of hemiplegia
- **d)** Postural hypotension is seen in Cushing's disease

45 Regarding anaemias
- **a)** Macrocytosis without megaloblastosis occurs in haemolytic anaemia
- **b)** Long-term treatment with Phenytoin sodium for epilepsy can cause megaloblastic anaemia
- **c)** The Schilling test is used to diagnose pernicious anaemia caused by folate deficiency
- **d)** Subacute combined degeneration of the spinal cord is caused by vitamin B12 deficiency

46 Regarding haemophilias
- **a)** They show autosomal recessive inheritance pattern
- **b)** The prothrombin time and bleeding time are prolonged
- **c)** Factor VIII levels less than 1% of normal are associated with severe frequent symptoms
- **d)** Christmas disease (haemophilia B) is caused by a deficiency of factor IX

47 The lesser sciatic foramen transmits the
- **a)** Nerve to the obturator externus
- **b)** Pudendal artery and nerve
- **c)** Inferior gluteal artery
- **d)** Obturator internus muscle and its nerve

48 The larynx
- **a)** Is bounded superiorly by the ary-epiglotiic folds
- **b)** In its interior mucosa is supplied by the recurrent laryngeal nerve up to the level of the vestibular fold
- **c)** Lies opposite the third to sixth cervical vertebrae

d) Gives attachment to muscles supplied by the first cervical nerve root

49 Regarding the nerves to the lower limb

a) They are all derived from both the lumbar and sacral plexus
b) The lumbar plexus passes through the substance of the psoas muscle
c) The femoral nerve arises from L1, 2 and 3
d) The femoral nerve terminates as the saphenous nerve to supply sensation to the medial aspect of the big toe

50 In evaluating study results

a) Confidence intervals provide more information than *p* values
b) A 95% confidence interval is the range at which the true value will be found 95% of the time
c) If the confidence interval crosses the line of zero difference then the results are statistically significant
d) A narrow confidence interval indicates the need for increasing the sample size to get valid results

Practice Paper 7

1 Regarding disorders of haemoglobin

a) Beta-chain variant haemoglobins are more common than alpha-chain variant haemoglobins

b) In the deoxygenated state, the solubility of Hb-S is 10 times than that of Hb-A

c) In β-thalassaemia major, foetal haemoglobin constitutes 10–98% of the total haemoglobin

d) Haemoglobin Bart's is the asymptomatic form of the α-thalassaemia gene

2 In treatment of coagulation disorders

a) Pyrogenic and allergic reactions can occur with plasma component infusions

b) Local pressure and topical application of adrenaline in bleeding wounds in patients with coagulation disorders is ineffective

c) Protamine sulphate can be used to treat bleeding during heparin therapy

d) After administration of vitamin K, the prothrombin takes up to 2 hours to normalise

3 The pancreas

a) Is mainly a retroperitoneal organ

b) The accessory duct opens in the duodenum just below the major duodenal papilla

c) Develops from both dorsal and ventral diverticula of the foregut

d) The superior mesenteric vessels lie anterior to the neck of the pancreas

4 Regarding facial X-rays

a) A tear drop sign is suggestive of an orbital floor fracture

b) Submentovertical projection is used to assess zygomatic arch fractures

c) One fracture of the mandible should raise the possibility of a second fracture on the opposite side
d) Nasal bone fractures are confirmed on plain radiographs of the nasal bones

5 The brachial plexus
a) The long thoracic nerve arises from the anterior divisions of the superior and middle trunks
b) The posterior cord contains contributions from all roots of the brachial plexus (C5–T1)
c) The musculocutaneous nerve which is a branch of the lateral cord supplies all three flexor muscles in the anterior compartment of the arm
d) The ulnar nerve is a terminal branch of the posterior cord

6 Regarding statistics
a) The ordinal scale involves ranking of the variable
b) The Mann–Whitney test is used in unmatched or independent samples
c) The experimental or research hypothesis is also known as the null hypothesis
d) In a positively skewed distribution the median is higher than the mean

7 Regarding chemical mediators in acute inflammation
a) Complement C3a is highly chemotactic to most leucocytes
b) Serotonin causes vasodilatation and increased vascular permeability
c) Nitric oxide activates platelet aggregation and adhesion
d) IL-1 and TNF induce systemic acute phase response such as fever

8 Warfarin
a) Is over 99% bound to plasma albumin
b) Should never be administered during pregnancy
c) Blocks the gama-carboxylation of factors VIII and II
d) Interacts with metronidazole inhibiting its metabolic transformation

9 Ibuprofen
a) Is extensively metabolised in the kidneys
b) Can cause pruritis, tinnitus and fluid retention as side effects

c) Is more than 99% protein-bound
d) Is contraindicated in patients with nasal polyps

10 Plasma hormones
a) Act by activating the cyclic AMP mechanism
b) React with a receptor substance on the cell membrane to activate specific genes
c) Include growth hormone which increases the transport of amino acids into certain cells
d) Can create specific messenger RNA molecules

11 The deep peroneal nerve
a) Supplies only some of the muscles of the anterior compartment of the lower leg
b) Has no cutaneous branches
c) Runs in company with the anterior tibial artery
d) Needs to be blocked to provide adequate anaesthesia of the sole of the foot

12 The parasympathetic nervous system
a) Has the vagus nerve as the largest contribution of its cranial outflow
b) Has the sacral outflow from S1, 2, 3
c) Has afferent fibres which are completely independent of them and do not relay in autonomic ganglia
d) When injured following a spinal cord injury can manifest as priapism

13 Regarding fluid and electrolyte balance
a) An 'average' person weighing 70 kg contains about 30 L of water in total
b) The extracellular fluid compartment is twice as large as the intracellular fluid compartment
c) Sodium ions make the highest contribution to total plasma osmolality
d) Normal GFR in males is about 130 mL/min

14 Regarding respiratory physiology
a) The intrapleural pressure is always negative in relation to the intra-alveolar pressure
b) Minute volume is the product of respiratory rate and the vital capacity

- **c)** Lung compliance is the change in respiratory pressure per unit change in lung volume
- **d)** Surfactant molecules are more in small alveoli than in larger alveoli

15 With hypothyroidism

- **a)** A goitre frequently occurs and contains large amounts of colloid substance
- **b)** Thyroid stimulating hormone (TSH) concentration is always very high
- **c)** Can result in generalised hyporeflexia
- **d)** If it is severe it can cause a marked bradycardia and even T wave inversion

16 Regarding CNS infections

- **a)** Negri bodies are found in CMV encephalitis
- **b)** *Cryptococcus neoformans* causes chronic meningitis
- **c)** *Borrelia burgdorferi* can cause aseptic meningitis
- **d)** Polio viruses have a propensity for the upper motor neurons in the spinal cord

17 Gonorrhoea

- **a)** Has an incubation period of 2–10 days
- **b)** May be asymptomatic in 10% of women
- **c)** Is a Gram-positive diplococcus
- **d)** Can cause ophthalmia neonatorum in babies born to infected mothers

18 The ascending aorta

- **a)** Has no branches
- **b)** Is related posteriorly to the left main bronchus
- **c)** Lies intrapericardially
- **d)** Is about 2 cm long and reaches as far as the right sternocalvicular joint

19 The urinary bladder

- **a)** Can be injured without an associated pelvic fracture
- **b)** Has no peritoneal covering
- **c)** Is attached to the umbilicus
- **d)** Is separated from the symphysis pubis by thick fibrous tissue

20 Regarding abnormal white cell counts

- **a)** Atypical, enlarged and pleomorphic lymphocytes are seen in viral hepatitis

- **b)** Propylthiouracil and carbimazole can induce severe neutrophilia
- **c)** Felty's syndrome is the association of chronic neutropenia with splenomegaly and rheumatoid arthritis
- **d)** High dose corticosteroid administration produces lymphopenia

21 Regarding polycythaemia rubra vera
- **a)** Most commonly presents between 20 and 40 years of age
- **b)** Overproduction of red cells and platelets is responsible for most of the morbidity and mortality
- **c)** Pruritus aggravated by a hot bath is an important symptom in diagnosis
- **d)** Venesection is a method of treatment when symptoms are distressing

22 Regarding systemic lupus erythematosus
- **a)** More common in females than males
- **b)** Detection of antinuclear antibodies is highly specific
- **c)** Acute necrotising vasculitis with fibrinoid deposits is typical
- **d)** The kidneys are rarely involved

23 Regarding antidiuretic hormone
- **a)** The posterior pituitary gland secretes antidiuretic hormone and oxytocin
- **b)** ADH is released in response to stimulation of the osmoreceptors in the supraoptic nucleus by a low concentration of sodium in the blood
- **c)** ADH increases water reabsorption in the distal tubule by increasing the pore size in the epithelial cells to allow water molecules to diffuse through
- **d)** ADH is released in massive quantities in response to severe stress such as operations or trauma

24 The heart rate is increased by
- **a)** Stimulation of pain fibres in the trigeminal nerve
- **b)** Inspiration
- **c)** Grief
- **d)** Increased activity of atrial stretch receptors

25 Distributive shock
- **a)** Due to endotoxins, glucocorticoids are of value
- **b)** Can be caused by a re-exposure to the same antigen of a previously sensitised individual

c) Is more severe in a febrile patient
d) Can occur when sudden autonomic activity results in vasoconstriction in blood vessels

26 Folliculitis
a) Is an inflammation of the ovarian follicle
b) The causative organism in the majority of cases is *Staph aureus*
c) Cephalosporins are effective in its treatment
d) Diagnosis depends on microbiological tests

27 The basal ganglia
a) Consists of the corpus striatum and claustrum only
b) Is divided by the posterior limb of the internal capsule
c) Has a lentiform nucleus which is made up of the putamen and the globus pallidus
d) May have lesions which cause all of the following: parkinsonism, Wilson's disease, chorea and athetosis

28 Regarding the ankle joint
a) This is purely a hinge joint
b) Inversion and eversion occur at the tibiotalar joint
c) In full dorsiflexion there is no laxity because the body of the talus is wider anteriorly
d) The deltoid ligament is the most commonly injured ligament in the ankle

29 Regarding the anatomy of the sensory transmission system
a) The sensory nerve fibres enter the spinal cord through the anterior roots of the spinal nerves
b) Some of the fibres divide and turn upwards in the dorsal columns and continue up to the medulla where the second synapse occurs
c) The fibres then course upwards through the brainstem in a column of fibres called the medial lemniscus and terminate in the thalamus
d) In the thalamus there is another synapse and then fibres pass through the internal capsule to the sensory cortex behind the central sulcus

30 Brain death is likely if all of the following are present
a) Decerebrate posturing
b) Fixed and dilated pupils

c) Absent brainstem reflexes
d) No spontaneous respiratory effort

31 Which of the following are true/false statements?
a) Summation is a true interaction
b) Pharmaceutical interactions can occur in vitro
c) Synergism of two drugs produce an effect greater than would have been expected
d) Potentiation is the enhancement of the effect of one drug by another

32 Glucagon
a) Is synthesised in the D cells of the pancreatic islets
b) Has a half-life similar to that of insulin
c) Has weak inotropic effects on the heart
d) Is used in treating severe hypoglycaemic reactions in type I diabetes

33 The following is true of skeletal muscle control
a) The muscle spindle and golgi tendon apparatus are both receptors
b) The muscle spindle and the golgi tendon apparatus transmit impulses to the spinal cord and occurs entirely at a subconscious level
c) The intrafusal muscle fibres are excited by a special type of motor nerve fibre called delta fibre
d) The middle of the muscle spindle contracts when stimulated and this is transmitted ultimately to the CNS to apprise it of the degree of contraction of muscles

34 The following areas of the brain take part in the planning and execution of a voluntary movement
a) The intermediate cerebellum
b) The basal ganglia
c) The premotor cortex
d) The lateral cerebellum

35 The coronary sinus
a) Receives venous blood from the venae cordis minimae
b) Receives venous blood from the anterior cardiac vein
c) Opens directly into the left atrium
d) Originates from the sinus venosus

36 The palatine tonsil
- **a)** Has a sensory innervation from the lesser palatine nerve
- **b)** Has its lymph drainage to the jugulodigastric node in the deep cervical chain of lymph nodes
- **c)** Is separated from the middle constrictor by the carotid sheath
- **d)** Is a derivative of the second pharyngeal pouch

37 Regarding randomisation
- **a)** Randomisation gives the best chance of matching the control and intervention group
- **b)** Tossing of a coin is an acceptable means of randomisation
- **c)** Computerised random-number generators lead to pseudo-randomisation
- **d)** Pseudo-randomisation precludes clinician concealment

38 About the FAB classification of acute leukaemias
- **a)** It is based on the various clinical features and the bone marrow morphology
- **b)** There are six different types of acute lymphoblastic leukaemia
- **c)** In erythroleukaemia, erythroblasts form more than 50% of marrow nucleated cells
- **d)** Leukaemia is classified as acute when more than 30% of bone marrow consists of blast cells

39 The following are causes of hematuria
- **a)** Schistosomiasis
- **b)** Urinary tract infection
- **c)** Renal papillary necrosis
- **d)** Glomerulonephritis

40 Factors that suggest increased suicide risk in a patient with overdose are
- **a)** Female
- **b)** Age group 20–40 years
- **c)** Separated, widowed or divorced
- **d)** Alcoholism

41 The following are true of the brainstem
- **a)** The dorsal surface of the pons forms part of the floor of the IVth ventricle
- **b)** The VIIth cranial nerve emerges from the junction between the pons and medulla

- **c)** The swellings on either side of the anteromedian groove of the medulla are formed by the pyramidal tracts
- **d)** It can be forced through the foramen magnum when there is a substantial rise in intracranial pressure and result in cardiorespiratory arrest

42 The right ovary
- **a)** Is covered by peritoneum in the adult
- **b)** Is drained by veins which terminates in the IVC
- **c)** When diseased can cause pain in the cutaneous distribution of the obturator nerve
- **d)** Has a blood supply from the abdominal aorta

43 Typhoid
- **a)** May present to the ED with profound fatigue and delirium
- **b)** Leucocytosis is common
- **c)** Chloramphenicol is a first-line drug used
- **d)** The incubation period is 7 days

44 Giardiasis
- **a)** Causes large intestinal disease
- **b)** Is the most common parasitic infection in travellers returning to the UK
- **c)** May present with passage of pale stools and steatorrhoea
- **d)** Can be excluded if the stool do not show cysts and trophozoites on microscopy

45 Prolonged administration of glucocorticoids results in
- **a)** Proximal myopathy
- **b)** Hypertension
- **c)** Hyperkalaemia
- **d)** Posterior sub-capsular cataract

46 Atracurium
- **a)** Is a non-depolarising neuromuscular blocking agent
- **b)** Is metabolised by the liver
- **c)** Has virtually no effect on the cardiovascular system
- **d)** Has a duration of action of about 20 minutes

47 When rising from the supine to the upright position
- **a)** Stroke volume drops by about 40%
- **b)** Total peripheral resistance rises by 25%

c) Cardiac output falls by 25%
d) Heart rate slows by about 25 beats per minute

48 With hearing
a) Movement of the handle of the malleus causes the stapes to move back and forth against the round window of the cochlea so transmitting sound waves to the cochlea fluid
b) The organ of Corti lies in the cochlea and is the receptor organ that generates nerve impulses in response to vibrations of the vestibular membrane
c) Vibrating hair cells excite the cochlear nerve by shearing back and forth against the tectorial membrane
d) Sound is transmitted from the cochlear nerve via the medial geniculate body to the auditory cortex which is located in the superior gyrus of the temporal lobe

49 The following is true of orthopaedic conditions
a) A Gamekeeper's thumb is the rupture of the ulnar collateral ligament of the proximal interphalangeal joint
b) Necrosis of the femoral head occurs in Perthe's disease
c) Kienbock's disease is an osteochondritis of the calcaneum
d) Osgood–Schlatter's disease is most common in athletic youngsters

50 In the Glasgow Coma Scale the following scores are true
a) Eye opening to speech scores 4 (four)
b) No verbal response scores 0 (zero)
c) Patient obeying commands scores 6 (six)
d) Flexion response to pain scores 2 (two)

Practice Paper 8

1 Cyclic AMP

a) Is cyclic 3′,6′ adenosine monophosphate

b) Can be formed intracellularly when the stimulating hormone binds to a specific receptor on the cell membrane

c) Adenyl cyclase is activated when the hormone binds to the membrane receptor

d) Adenyl cyclase converts adenosine diphosphate into cyclic AMP

2 Intracranial pressure

a) Is more important than cerebral perfusion pressure in the management of head injuries

b) Is mean arterial pressure – cerebral perfusion pressure

c) Is normally 20 mm Hg

d) Can be maintained at normal levels even with an expanding intracranial mass by displacing both CSF and cerebral venous blood from the cranium

3 The pulse

a) May be collapsing in type in pregnancy

b) Is slow rising in mitral stenosis

c) Is jerky in severe mitral regurgitation

d) Is paradoxical (pulsus paradoxus) in severe asthma

4 Typical findings in DKA include

a) Peripheral blood leucocytosis

b) Decreased serum K^+ at presentation

c) Arterial blood gases: $PaO_2 = 7$ kPa, $PaCO_2 = 7$ kPa, $HCO_3 = 23$ mmol/L, pH $= 7.20$

d) A water deficit of 5–10 L

5 Regarding nematode infections

a) *Brugia malayi* is transmitted by the anopheles mosquito

b) *Dracunculus medinensis* is transmitted by ingestion of water containing infected cyclops

c) Cutaneous larva migrans can be treated with Diethylcarbamazine
d) *Ascaris lumbricoides* can cause acute appendicitis

6 In the hand
a) The dorsal interossei cause abduction of index, middle and ring fingers at the metacarpophalangeal joints
b) The median nerve innervates all the lumbrical muscles of the hand
c) The cephalic vein originates from the medial side of the dorsal venous arch
d) The only part of the radial nerve that enters the hand is the superficial branch

7 The gastrointestinal tract
a) The duodenum has the widest lumen of the small intestine
b) The lesser omentum is attached to the lesser curvature
c) Meckel's diverticulum is present in 20% of the population
d) The duodenojejunal flexure is surrounded by the ligamentum teres

8 Acid–base physiology
a) Normal hydrogen ion concentration is between 35 and 45 nmol/L
b) Haemoglobin acts as a buffer with high capacity to bind hydrogen ions
c) The normal anion gap is 20–30 mmol/L
d) A high anion gap is caused by rise in plasma bicarbonate

9 Regarding hyponatraemia
a) SIADH can be seen in pneumonia
b) Hyponatraemia is present despite sodium retention in cardiac failure
c) Cushing's syndrome causes hyponatraemia due to sodium loss
d) Intravenous infusion of 0.9% NaCl is always needed to correct hyponatraemia due to diarrhoea

10 The following drugs should not be used to treat an acute attack of gout
a) Aspirin
b) Colchicine
c) Allopurinol
d) Indomethacin

11 Sulphonylureas
- **a)** Can produce hypoglycaemia
- **b)** Tend to produce weight loss
- **c)** Act by increasing insulin release
- **d)** Can rarely cause thrombocytopenia

12 The following is true about the retina
- **a)** Rods and cones in the retina transform light energy into neuronal signals
- **b)** The rods are responsible for colour vision
- **c)** The cones provide greater acuity of vision than rods because one cone is connected to one optic nerve fibre
- **d)** Almost all colour blind people are male because the colour genes are found in the female sex chromosome

13 Tendons
- **a)** Carry tensile forces from muscle to bone
- **b)** Contain type I collagen fibrils
- **c)** Get its blood supply from periosteal insertion
- **d)** Do not adapt to changes in their mechanical environment

14 Arteries in the upper limb
- **a)** The profunda brachii artery is a branch of the third part of the axillary artery
- **b)** The common interosseous artery in the forearm is a branch of the radial artery
- **c)** The ulnar artery leaves the cubital fossa by passing deep to the pronator teres muscle
- **d)** Allen's test is used to test for adequacy of anastomoses between the radial and ulnar arteries

15 The right coronary artery
- **a)** Occlusion results in anterior infarction
- **b)** Provides a posterior descending branch which runs in the AV groove
- **c)** Usually provides an atrioventricular nodal branch
- **d)** Occlusion does not affect the right ventricle

16 Regarding a diagnostic test
- **a)** Specificity is the proportion of true negatives correctly identified by the test
- **b)** Sensitivity is the proportion of people with the disease who react positively to the test

- **c)** Positive predictive value is the proportion of those who test positive and who actually do not have the disease
- **d)** Negative predictive value is the proportion of those who test negative and who do actually have the disease

17 Regarding haemolytic anaemias

- **a)** The absence of jaundice excludes the diagnosis of haemolytic anaemia
- **b)** Plasma haptoglobin level is usually reduced in haemolytic disease
- **c)** In haemolytic disorders the reticulocyte count ranges from 5 to 20%
- **d)** The presence of spherocytes on a peripheral blood film is diagnostic of hereditary spherocytosis

18 With abnormal growth hormone secretion

- **a)** Failure of the pituitary to secrete growth hormone results in dwarfism
- **b)** Gigantism is almost always caused by excessive secretion of growth hormone due to dysfunction of the hypothalamus before adolescence
- **c)** Acromegaly is due to a growth hormone secreting tumour developing after adolescence and results in enlargement of the nose, lips, tongue and liver
- **d)** Acromegaly causes disproportionate growth of the mandible, hands, feet and sternum

19 Regarding medicolegal issues

- **a)** Where possible always seek patient's full, informed consent in 'not for resuscitation' decision
- **b)** The Research Ethics Committee do not have lay membership
- **c)** A mistake in making the correct diagnosis amounts to medical negligence
- **d)** Patient's confidentiality can be relaxed in cases of statutory disclosure

20 Regarding the eye and the orbit

- **a)** The optic nerve and the ophthalmic artery pass through the optic canal
- **b)** The levator palpebrae superioris is an elevator of the eyeball
- **c)** The lateral rectus is supplied by the sixth cranial nerve
- **d)** The aqueous humour drains into the canal of Schlemm at the angle of the anterior chamber

21 The prostate gland

a) Is palpable on rectal examination despite transection of the puboprostatic ligaments

b) Drains via its venous plexus to the internal vertebral plexus of veins

c) Lies against the inferior fascia of the urogenital diaphragm

d) Is traversed by the vasa deferentia

22 Malaria

a) Symptoms occasionally may not develop for 12 months or more

b) Diagnosis is based on demonstration of parasites in a single thin film

c) Respiratory distress, absent corneal reflexes, fits or Hb of <5 g/dL indicates a poor prognosis

d) Treatment of choice is with chloroquine for *P. falciparum*

23 Infective endocarditis

a) Can occur with many different organisms and include fungi

b) *Streptococcus viridans* is one of the commoner organisms

c) Typically occurs in patients with abnormal or prosthetic valves but also in those with congenital heart defects such as VSD or PDA

d) Is often easily diagnosed due to new advances in echocardiography

24 Drug interactions may result

a) From competition for plasma protein binding sites

b) From displacement for tissue binding sites

c) In an additive or synergistic response

d) From pharmacokinetic mechanisms alone

25 Diclofenac

a) Is a highly selective cyclo-oxygenase inhibitor

b) Accumulates in the synovial fluid

c) Its clearance is influenced by renal dysfunction

d) May cause elevation of serum aminotransferases

26 Regarding the following disease states

a) Chorea is due to damage of the globus pallidus

b) Athetosis occurs when a person performs one pattern of movement for a few seconds and then suddenly jump to an entirely new pattern

c) Hemiballismus is an uncontrollable succession of violent movements of large areas of the body and is due to injury to the subthalamus
d) In full blown Parkinson's disease a person walks in a crouch like an ape but with tense muscles

27 The control of blood pressure
a) Is mainly due to activity in the vasomotor area of the midbrain
b) Is influenced by the discharge of the baroreceptors in the aortic arch
c) Is defective in patients with hypoaldosteronism
d) Is not influenced by a high pCO_2

28 The following is true of hernias
a) Direct inguinal hernias commonly strangulate
b) An irreducible hernia may be asymptomatic
c) Malgaigne's bulge is a normal clinical finding
d) A saphena varix is a type of femoral hernia

29 Regarding the following conditions
a) Ludwig's angina is a cellulitis of the sublingual and submandibular spaces
b) Fournier's gangrene is an acute inflammatory oedema of the nose
c) Herpes zoster ophthalmicus results from an infection of the trigeminal ganglion
d) Erythema ab igne is seen in streptococcal cellulitis

30 Regarding lymphomas
a) Reed–Sternberg cells are giant cells with large round nucleus and prominent eosinophilic nucleoli
b) The presence of well-differentiated cells and nodular growth pattern in non-Hodgkin's lymphoma is associated with more favourable prognosis
c) Staging of the disease is essential to design an appropriate treatment plan
d) Doxorubicin can be used in the treatment of non-Hodgkin's lymphoma

31 Regarding the coagulation mechanism
a) Factors II, V, VII, and IX are vitamin K-dependent coagulation factors

b) Plasminogen activator is present in urine
c) Antithrombin III inhibits factor Xa
d) In the classical 'intrinsic' system factor Xa is formed by the proteolytic activation of factor X by factor XIa

32 The superficial inguinal lymph nodes may be enlarged due to pathology in the
a) Lateral portion of the uterine (fallopian) tube
b) Vagina
c) Body of the uterus
d) Anal canal above the pectinate line

33 The posterior triangle of the neck
a) Contains the trunks of the brachial plexus
b) Contains the suprascapular nerve
c) The accessory nerve (XIth cranial nerve) runs between the two layers of fascia
d) The inferior belly of the omohyoid muscle crosses its floor

34 The intercostal spaces
a) Are traversed by posterior intercostal arteries that give branches to the spinal cord
b) Has the internal intercostal muscle which runs downwards and forwards reaching the costochondral junction anteriorly
c) May tract pus originating from the thoracic vertebrae and point in the mid-axillary line
d) Are traversed by intercostal veins which drain mainly into the azygous and hemiazygous veins

35 The following are measures of dispersion
a) Average
b) Standard deviation
c) Median
d) Mean deviation

36 Regarding transplantation
a) Infections with HLA cross-reactive organisms can sensitise the recipient to antigens in the graft causing hyperacute rejection
b) Acute cellular rejection does not respond to immunosuppressive therapy
c) Acute rejection occurs within a few days of transplantation
d) Subacute vasculitis produces bouts of clinical rejection

37 Local anaesthetics

a) Are usually injected in an acid solution and are soluble in water
b) Act by causing sodium channel blockade
c) May cause systemic toxicity which manifests itself initially as convulsions and arrhythmias
d) Have different toxic doses and the least toxic is lignocaine

38 Steroids for the management of asthma

a) Work by reducing the hyposensitivity of the airways
b) Must be tapered in dose after a 5-day course of oral prednisolone
c) Have minimal systemic absorption when used as inhaled aerosol therapy
d) Causes oropharyngeal candidiasis when steroid inhalers are used

39 Regarding aldosterone

a) It is secreted mainly by the zona reticularis of the adrenal cortex
b) Sodium reabsorption by aldosterone takes several hours to occur because it has to activate a genetic mechanism
c) It also causes reabsorption of chloride ions from the renal tubules
d) It causes a large increase in cardiac output

40 The piriformis muscle

a) Is attached to the lesser trochanter
b) Exits the pelvis through the lesser sciatic foramen
c) Is a lateral rotator of the hip
d) Has the sciatic nerve emerging superior to its upper border

41 The femoral nerve

a) Lies one fingerbreadth lateral to the femoral artery at the level of the inguinal ligament
b) Gives motor branches to the quadriceps, sartorius and pectineus muscles
c) Gives off the lateral cutaneous nerve of the thigh
d) Is easily blocked with local anaesthetic and provides substantial pain relief for patients with a fractured neck of femur

42 Regarding osmolarity

a) Osmolarity is the number of osmoles per kilogram of solvent
b) Osmolality is the number of osmoles per litre of solution
c) Plasma osmolality should be higher than the calculated osmolarity

d) Urinary osmolarity should always be measured in preference to urinary osmolality

43 Denervated skeletal muscle may display

a) Paralysis

b) Atrophy

c) Increased sensitivity to acetylcholine

d) Fibrillations

44 Regarding cranial nerve examination

a) In the corneal reflex the efferent limb is the trigeminal nerve

b) Bell's phenomenon is seen in upper motor neuron lesions of the VIIth cranial nerve

c) Rinne's test determines whether air conduction is better than bone conduction

d) The gag reflex is determined by the Xth and XIth cranial nerves

45 *Chlamydia trachomatis*

a) Is the most commonly reported bacterial sexually transmitted disease

b) Has an incubation period of 3–6 weeks

c) Is asymptomatic in as many as 80% of women

d) Is the commonest cause of epididymitis in men over the age of 35

46 Regarding the knee joint

a) The anterior cruciate ligament attaches to the anterior aspect of the femur

b) The stability of the knee relies on the surrounding muscles rather than the ligaments

c) The collateral ligaments are injured with the knee in full extension

d) The menisci are injured when the knee is in some degree of flexion

47 In the pelvis the following structures lie between ureter and peritoneum

a) The superior vesicle artery

b) The vas deferens in the male

c) The obturator nerve

d) The uterine artery in the female

48 In hereditary haemorrhagic telangiectasia

a) Haematuria is the most common symptom

b) Hypochromic microcytic anaemia is common

c) Platelet count is commonly reduced
d) The skin lesions are seen mostly on the chest and abdomen

49 Regarding platelet production
a) Each megakaryocyte produces about 1000 platelets
b) The lifespan of platelets in circulation is about 80–100 days
c) The normal platelet count ranges between 50 and 100 × 10^9/L
d) Platelets have round or oval nucleus with closely clumped chromatin

50 Regarding acute inflammation
a) Exudate is an inflammatory extravascular fluid with a specific gravity of <1.012
b) The intravascular osmotic pressure is elevated
c) Interleukin 1 and tumour necrosis factor induce the synthesis of adhesion molecules on the endothelium
d) Arachidonic acid metabolites act as chemotactic agents for neutrophils

Answers

Paper 1 Answers

1 T F T F (The superior mesenteric vein drains blood from the ascending and transverse colon via the ileocolic, right colic and middle colic veins. The right and left gastric veins are tributaries to the portal vein.)
2 F T F F (The frontal bone articulates with the parietal bone at the coronal suture. The zygomatic arch is formed by the zygomatic process of the temporal bone and the temporal process of the zygomatic bone. The optic nerve passes through the optic canal.)
3 F T T T (They are carried in very large nerve fibres.)
4 F F T F (Moderate changes in environmental temperature do not lead to a change in cardiac output, but high environmental temperature increases cardiac output. Standing from a lying down position decreases the cardiac output and so does rapid arrhythmias.)
5 F T T T (It is dissolved in distilled water.)
6 F F T F (Aspirin has no effect on mast cells, it however stabilises lysosomes, inhibits the migration of polymorphonuclear leucocytes and macrophages into sites of inflammation.)
7 F T T T
8 F F F T (All forms of shock increases plasma renin activity, standing quietly reduces blood pressure causing an increase in plasma renin activity.)
9 T F T F (The intervertebral foramina are formed by notches in the pedicles. Spina bifida occurs when the two centres in the arch do not fuse posteriorly.)
10 T F F F (The mitral valve guards the left AV orifice and its anterior cusp is larger than the posterior. Both cusps are anchored by tendinous cord to the papillary muscles.)
11 T T T T
12 T F T F (Haemoglobin makes up about 90% of the dry weight of the red blood cell. Red blood cells carry 100 times the amount of oxygen that can be carried in plasma alone.)

13 F T F F (Vomiting is an active process and requires a reasonable degree of consciousness. Passive regurgitation is what can happen at any time. A large number of patients do not require HDU, e.g. stroke patients do better on a Stroke Unit, patients requiring palliative care etc. Patients not requiring CT head = obvious poisoning; postictal patients where there is no concern about intracranial pathology.)

14 T T F T (Do not provide a written police statement before patient consent is obtained.)

15 F T F T (Only the posterior 1/3 has no papillae. Palatoglossus is NOT supplied by the hypoglossal nerve but by cranial nerve XI.)

16 F F T F (The aortic opening is at T12, the IVC travels through the central tendon and when paralysed is elevated on X-ray.)

17 T T F T (A normal chest X-ray in a symptomatic patient does not exclude tuberculosis.)

18 T F T T (PID includes endometriosis, salpingitis, oophoritis and peritonitis. There is a five times risk of developing ectopic pregnancy with PID.)

19 T T T T (Heparin and protamine interaction is an example of chemical antagonism.)

20 T F F F (Cimetidine inhibits the P450 enzyme in the liver. Calcium-channel blockers increase the plasma concentration of midazolam and digoxin. β-blocker concentration is increased when used with cimetidine.)

21 T F F F (A rise in intracellular osmolality stimulates the secretion of ADH. Aldosterone increases sodium reabsorption and therefore reduces excretion. Renin is secreted in response to decreases in blood pressure.)

22 T F T F (The precordial leads in an athlete's ECG may show prominent J waves and deep, narrow Q waves. A systolic load displays an ST depression – strain pattern. A sternal fracture causing a myocardial contusion is a likely cause of an ST segment elevation on an ECG.)

23 T T F T (History and examination alone cannot safely exclude a deep vein thrombosis. If a DVT is suspected, further investigations are needed.)

24 T T F F (Full thickness burns are not painful. They have no sensation. Alkalis are more destructive and penetrate more deeply than acids.)

25 T F T T (Fanconi's anaemia is familial aplastic anaemia and does not give rise to megaloblasts.)

26 F F T T (It is usually a sporadic illness and does not spread in an epidemic manner. Slight-to-moderate splenomegaly occurs in more than 40% of cases.)

27 T F T T (The hip is also innervated by the obturator nerve.)

28 T T T T

29 F F F F (The ureter is a lateral relation of the lateral vaginal fornix and is supported laterally by the cardinal ligaments. Its posterior relation is the rectovaginal pouch of Douglas.)

30 T T F F (Approximately, 95% of the values will lie between two standard deviations from the mean. The mean is the best measure of central tendency in a normal distribution.)

31 T F F T (T lymphocytes constitute 60–70% of the lymphocytes circulating in blood. IgG is the most abundant of circulating immunoglobulins.)

32 F T F T (Sodium nitrite is used for cyanide, although hydroxocobalamin, sodium thiocyanate and dicobalt edetate may also be used; calcium gluconate gel is used for hydrofluoric acid burns.)

33 T F T F (Nitrous oxide is a powerful analgesic especially when combined with volatile anaesthetic. With the reduction in pain it reduces tachycardia and increased BP indirectly.)

34 T F T F (Thyroxine remains stored in the follicle still part of the thyroglobulin molecule before being released into the blood where it immediately binds to a plasma protein. It is released from this protein over a period of days so thyroxine is slowly released to tissues; it can only double the body's metabolic rate.)

35 F F T T (The ulnar nerve passes behind the medial epicondyle of the humerus. The extensor pollicis longus forms the medial border of the anatomical snuff box.)

36 T F T F (A gap of 5 mm or more at the symphysis is a fracture of the symphysis. A fracture at one point of the 'ring' is associated frequently with a second fracture elsewhere in the 'ring'.)

37 F F T F ('a' waves occur with atrial systole and absent in atrial fibrillation. Giant 'v' waves are seen in tricuspid regurgitation due to an increase in passive filling of the right atrium. Kussmaul's sign is when the JVP rises with inspiration and is due to constrictive pericarditis, restrictive cardiomyopathy, pericardial tamponade and right heart failure.)

38 F T F T (Antigravity reflexes are integrated in the medulla and proprioceptors in the distal flexors cause a positive supporting reaction.)

39 T T F T (Only minute quantities of mineralocorticoid are required.)

40 T T F T (Tetanus is caused by the exotoxin produced by *Clostridium tetani*, the spores of which live in the soil and faeces. Tetanospasmin acts on both α and δ motor systems at synapses, resulting in disinhibition, the end result being marked flexor muscle spasm and autonomic dysfunction.)

41 T F F T (The typical viral causative agent is Coxsackie B; only occasionally is severe enough to cause heart failure.)

42 T F F T (It communicates with the deep veins with only two or three perforating veins. It has three tributaries at the groin = superficial epigastric, superficial circumflex iliac, superficial external pudendal veins.)

43 F F T T (The cutaneous nerves have afferent somatic fibres of general sensation and efferent autonomic fibres for the sweat gland, sebaceous glands and smooth muscle of hair and blood vessels. The nails grow slowly in immobilised limbs.)

44 T F F T (Proportion of immature cells is small as compared to acute leukaemia. Most cases can be distinguished from leukaemia on careful consideration of the clinical and haematological features. Marrow aspiration and trephine biopsy are usually diagnostic but not always needed.)

45 T T T T

46 F T F T (Wound healing involves chemotaxis, cell division, neovascularisation; synthesis of extracellular matrix and formation and remodelling of the scar. Activation of growth factors and other inflammatory mediators and orderly cell division without mutations is the key to healing.)

47 F T F T (The anion gap here is 41. There is moderate respiratory compensation, as the patient has to be hyperventilating to achieve a $PaCO_2$ of 3.9 kPa.)

48 T T F T (Tension pneumothorax impedes venous return.)

49 F T T T (Erythropoietin deficiency causes normocytic normochromic anaemia.)

50 T T T T

Paper 2 Answers

1 T T F T (The skin is often flushed and diaphoretic.)

2 T F F F (In suspected epiglottitis examination of the throat should be performed only by medical personnel experienced in intubation of small children. The peak incidence of acute bronchiolitis is between 3 and 6 months. Acute epiglottitis is caused by *H. influenza* type B bacterium and does require antibiotic therapy.)

3 F T F F (The ulnar nerve passes superficial to the flexor retinaculum, lies lateral to the tendon of flexor carpi ulnaris at the wrist. Clawing is most pronounced in the little and ring fingers as the lumbricals of the lateral two digits are supplied by the median nerve.)

4 T F F T (The pelvic splanchnic nerves also carry preganglionic parasympathetic fibres from sacral spinal cord S2–S4. Referred pain from midgut organs is felt in the umbilical region via spinal cord levels T9 and T10.)

5 T T T T

6 T T F T (The reticulocyte is slightly bigger in volume and diameter than the mature red cell.)

7 T T T F (You should not end a relationship with a patient solely because of a complaint the patient has made about you or your team.)

8 F T T F (SIRS can be diagnosed when two or more of the following are present. Pulse >90/min, temperature >38°C or <36°C, respiratory rate >20/min and WBC count <4,000/mm^3 or >12,000/mm^3.)

9 F T T T (It forms the floor of the third ventricle.)

10 F F T T (The symphysis pubis is a secondary cartilaginous joint which is a union between bones whose articular surfaces are covered with a thin lamina of hyaline cartilage. It is never lined with synovial membrane.)

11 T F F T (Chronic mucocutaneous candidiasis is a term used to describe a heterogeneous group of *Candida* infections of the skin, mucous membranes, hair and nails, which has a protracted course despite typical therapy. It is associated with T-cell lymphocyte dysfunction. Candidal pneumonia occurs rarely as bronchopneumonia and more commonly as nodular diffuse infiltrate.)

12 T T T F

13 F F F F (Carbamazepine increases clearance of other anticonvulsants. Valproate has no effect on sodium conductance but increases concentrations of GABA in the brain. Diplopia and ataxia are common side effects of carbamazepine and phenytoin. Hirsutism occurs to some degree in most patients on phenytoin.)

14 F T F F (There are four common antimicrobial mechanisms and these also include inhibition of protein synthesis and inhibition of nucleic acid synthesis. Some β-lactams are protected by a methoxy or other groups, e.g. methicillin. Tetracyclines act by inhibiting protein synthesis.)

15 T T T F (Stretching of the atrial stretch receptors by an increased venous return causes the heart rate to increase.)

16 F T T F (The protein in bone matrix is mostly type I collagen. It has a total blood flow of 200–400 mL/min. Bone crystal is made mostly of hydroxyapatites – $Ca_{10}(PO_4)_6\ (OH)_2$, sodium and small amounts of magnesium. It has a readily exchangeable pool of about 100 mmols of calcium.)

17 F F F T (Intubation may be avoided if the cause for unconsciousness is anticipated to reverse or be brief, e.g. hypoglycaemia, opiate poisoning and postictal phase. Another cause for hypotension must always be sought as raised ICP never causes hypotension.)

18 F T F F (Trauma to the first rib usually affects the trunks. Nerve avulsions and disruption require many months of dedicated rehabilitation for even a small amount of function to return.)

19 T T T T

20 F T T F (Thrombasthenia is a congenital qualitative platelet defect with deficiency of glycoprotein IIb/IIIa receptor in the membrane. The platelet count is normal. There is a 75–90% response rate to splenectomy in chronic ITP.)

21 T F T F (It divides into the anterior and posterior tibial arteries at the level of the lower border of popliteus muscle.)

22 T F F F (The SA node is supplied by the right coronary artery in over 55% of the population. The acute marginal branch arises from the right coronary artery. The right coronary artery also gives rise to the posterior interventricular artery in 85–90% of cases.)

23 F F F T (The spinal cord occupies the whole canal at 3 months of foetal life and at birth is at the level of L3. It finishes at the level of the disc between L1 and L2 and the filum terminale attaches to the coccyx.)

24 F F T T (Sensitivity = 90/(90 + 10), specificity = 105/(5 + 105), positive likelihood ratio = sensitivity/1 − specificity, negative likelihood ration = 1 − sensitivity/specificity.)

25 T T F T (Primary healing of a wound occurs when it is closed within 12–24 hours of its creation, e.g. clean surgical wound.)

26 T F T T (Because the organs of elimination can only clear the drug from the blood or plasma in direct contact with the organ, this blood or plasma is in equilibrium with the total volume of distribution. Hence, the time course of drug in the body will depend on both the volume of distribution and the clearance.)

27 F T T T (Atropine is an antimuscarinic drug and it has a bronchodilator action on the smooth muscles of the respiratory system.)

28 F T F F (The whole body potassium is low. Serum potassium is elevated due to extravasation of potassium from intracellular to extracellular compartment. The increased respiratory rate is actually trying to correct the metabolic acidosis by blowing off more CO_2. In hyperosmolar non-ketotic coma there is some amount of background insulin production and the insulin requirement is lower than in DKA.)

29 T F T T (The weakest portion of the clavicle is the middle third.)

30 T T T F (The epiphysis of the fifth metatarsal runs in the same longitudinal direction of the metatarsals whilst a fracture is always transverse.)

31 T F T T (The sodium ions flow to the inside of the fibre.)

32 F T T F (The amine, dopamine and serotonin penetrate the blood–brain barrier to a very limited degree, but their corresponding acid precursors (L-dopa and 5HT) enter the brain with ease. The blood–brain barrier is immature at birth, hence the syndrome of kernicterus in severe jaundice of the new born.)

33 F T F F (Injury to the long thoracic nerve causes winging of the scapula. The sciatic nerve is a branch of the sacral plexus. It is the largest nerve in the body and arises from five roots – L4, 5 and S1, 2 and 3. The diaphragm is supplied by the phrenic nerve – C3, 4 and 5. Injuries below this level will permit the patients to breathe.)

34 F T T T (Schistosomules mature into adult worms in the liver.)

35 T T F F (The infective period in chicken pox starts two days before the onset of rash. Epstein Barr virus is considered to be the cause of oral hairy leukoplakia.)

36 T F F T (The anterior jugular vein opens into the external jugular vein which in turn enters the subclavian vein. The origin of the internal jugular vein is the continuation of the sigmoid sinus.)

37 F F T F (The external auditory canal is only 3.5 cm long and only the outer 1/3 is cartilaginous. On using an auroscope one cannot see the stapes at all and only part of the incus.)

38 T T F F (Lupus anticoagulant predisposes to a thrombotic tendency in vivo. This antibody found in SLE is called 'anticoagulant' because it causes prolongation of PT and APTT. Platelet aggregation is prevented by inhibition of platelet cyclo-oxygenase by agents such as aspirin.)

39 T T F T (Transfusion haemosiderosis does not occur in patients who require repeated transfusion due to blood loss.)

40 T F T F (Mobility at fracture site interferes with and prevents subperiosteal new bone formation. Remodelling of bone is better in children than in adults.)

41 F T F T (The normal BMR is 60–70 calories per hour. Very high temperatures only increase BMR by twice the basal level.)

42 T F T T (The normal QRS duration is up to 120 milliseconds.)

43 F F T T (Potassium ranges from 3.5 to 5.0 mmol/L. Bilirubin ranges from 2 to 17 μmol/L.)

44 F F F T (HIV testing should not be offered in the ED and patients requesting the test should be referred to local infectious disease/GU units. IgG antibodies to HIV provide the evidence of infection. IgG antibodies may not appear until 3 months after exposure.)

45 F F F T (The gallbladder fossa is devoid of visceral peritoneum. The quadrate lobe has the gallbladder fossa to its right and the caudate lobe has the groove for the inferior vena cava to its right. The subphrenic and hepatorenal recesses are parts of the peritoneal cavity and are therefore continuous anteriorly.)

46 T T T T

47 T F F T (Due to blood loss the arterial baroreceptors are stretched to a lesser degree and sympathetic discharge increases. Vasoconstriction is most marked in the skin causing pallor and coolness and in the kidney leading to a decrease in urine output.)

48 T F F F (A small amount of albumin up to 25 mg/24 hours is found normally in the urine. Parathyroid hormone promotes phosphate excretion.)

49 F F T T (Pharmacokinetics is the science of the relationship between the movement of a drug through the body and the process affecting it.)

50 T T T F

Paper 3 Answers

1 T T T F (A proportion of blast cells of 30% or more is essential on the bone marrow for the diagnosis of acute leukaemia.)

2 T T F F (The ST elevation in chest leads should be at least 2 mm or more. Thrombolysis can be initiated up to 12 hours from the onset of chest pain.)

3 T T T T

4 T F F T (The cranial venous sinuses eventually drain into the internal jugular vein. The subarachnoid space is between the arachnoid and the pia mater.)

5 T T T T

6 T F T F (Kissing contacts are those where exchange of saliva is possible. Health care staff involved in patient care other than those who have given mouth-to-mouth resuscitation to the index case do not require chemoprophylaxis.)

7 F T T F (Pruritus ani is usually the only symptom in threadworm infection caused by *Enterobius vermicularis*. *Trichuris trichiura* does not pass through lungs.)

8 T F T F (Almost all benzodiazepines have active metabolites with CNS depressant effects. Diazepam has an elimination half-life between 50 and 150 hours.)

9 F F F T (The majority of drugs administered orally are absorbed by passive diffusion in the small intestine. Most of the peptides are broken down enzymatically before absorption.)

10 F T F T (Physiological dead space is the sum of anatomical dead space and alveolar dead space. $PaCO_2$ is the best indicator of alveolar ventilation.)

11 F T F F (In diabetes insipidus the urine:plasma osmolality is <1. In type II renal tubular acidosis the capacity to reabsorb bicarbonate in the proximal tubule is reduced. A total of 99% of the glomerular filtrate is reabsorbed in the renal tubules.)

12 F F T T

13 F T T F (Cullen's sign is not seen in acute appendicitis. It is a discolouration around the umbilicus seen in haemorrhagic pancreatitis. Psoas' test in acute appendicitis elicits pain on hyperextension of right hip.)

14 T T T T

15 T F T T (Sickling is readily demonstrated by the sickle test and the haemoglobin solubility test is positive in sickle-cell trait.)

16 T F T F (The aorta bifurcates at the level of L4 vertebra. The spleen extends from rib 9 to 11 and follows the contour of rib 10 from superior pole of the left kidney to just posterior to the mid-axillary line.)

17 F F T F (The pronator teres is supplied by the median nerve. The flexor pollicis longus originates from the anterior surface of the radius and adjacent half of the anterior surface of the interosseous membrane. Anconeus is the most medial of the superficial muscles in the posterior compartment.)

18 F F T F (The lateral boundary of the femoral triangle is the medial border of sartorius. The femoral artery and vein are contained within the femoral sheath. The neck of the femoral hernia is always lateral to the pubic tubercle.)

19 T T T T

20 F F F T (Wound healing is impaired by a poor blood supply to the wound and a poor venous drainage from the wound. Increased skin tension caused by tight sutures and the presence of infection, foreign bodies and necrotic tissue are other local factors that impede healing.)

21 T F F F (Has a half-life of 5–10 seconds; dipyridamole inhibits adenosine breakdown so the dose of adenosine has to be reduced. It has no place in rate control of AF but can be used to slow the rate of a regular narrow-complex tachycardia to determine whether atrial flutter is present.)

22 T T F T (Metformin should not be prescribed for patients with renal impairment, liver disease, alcoholism, uncontrolled cardiac failure and severe pulmonary insufficiency.)

23 T T T T

24 F T F T (Fasciculus cuneatus is lateral to the medial fasciculus gracilis. There are two motor tracts and one, the anterior cerebrospinal or direct pyramidal tract, descends without decussating in the medulla.)

25 T F T F (The first permanent tooth is at 6. The periodontal membrane appears as a radiolucent line around the root of each tooth.)

26 F T F T (pH ranges from 7.35 to 7.45, normal pO_2 ranges from 10.5 to 13.5.)

27 F T F F (Glucose is more than half of blood glucose in viral meningitis. Tuberculous meningitis has more mononuclear cells than polymorphs in CSF and CSF protein in bacterial meningitis is raised to 0.5–2.0 g/L.)

28 T T T T (Herpes zoster affecting lower thoracic segments can present as abdominal pain. Pleurisy involving the diaphragmatic pleura can present as abdominal pain.)

29 T T F T (Hepatitis B vaccination at birth to all babies whose mothers are Hep B positive.)

30 F F F T (The incubation period is 9–90 days. The enlarged lymph nodes are typically non-tender. Skin granulomas occur in the tertiary stage – mucous patches on the genitalia or mouth is the other cardinal sign of the secondary stage.)

31 T F F F (The superior rectal vein is a tributary of the inferior mesenteric vein. The rectum begins in front of the third sacral vertebra and its upper third is covered by peritoneum in its front and sides, its middle third on its front only and its lower third is embedded in the pelvic fascia.)

32 F T F F (The left phrenic nerve arises from the ventral rami of the third, fourth and fifth cervical nerves and descends in the mediastinum covered by the mediastinal pleura. It pierces the dome of the left diaphragm and gives branches to its under surface.)

33 T T T T

34 F T F T (The majority of cases of HDN are due to ABO incompatibility but cases due to Rh incompatibility are more severe. The maternal antibodies that cross the placenta are IgG antibodies.)

35 F T T F (In type 1 fracture there is a transverse fracture through the epiphyseal plate or physis. The width of the epiphyseal plate may be increased. In type 4 fracture the fracture line passes through all three elements of the bone – epiphysis, physis and metaphysis.)

36 T T T T

37 T T F T (The crossed extensor reflex involves a flexor reflex in one limb causing an extensor reflex in the opposite limb.)

38 F F T F (Release of local Thromboxane A2 occurs activating the coagulation cascade and contracting the bleeding vessels. ADH is released from the posterior pituitary. The basal vagal tone is decreased due to regulation of the baroreceptors.)

39 F T T T (Wounds heavily contaminated with soil and faecal matter (farm land), animal bite wounds, wounds over 6 hours old and those with devitalised tissue are prone to tetanus infection.)

40 F F F T (The internal urethral orifice in the male is the site of the involuntary sphincter, but it is a wide open canal that leads to the prostatic urethra. The navicular fossa is a dilatation just inside the very narrow external orifice. The colliculus seminalis is the most dilatable region of the urethra.)

41 T T T T

42 F F T F (It is a continuation of the external iliac artery and is located at the mid-inguinal point = midpoint between ASIS and the pubic symphysis (not pubic tubercle). It is very rarely injured by closed fractures of the shaft.)

43 T T T T

44 T T F T (The synovium lining joints, tendons and bursae are structurally identical. The surface of the synovium is permeable to water, small molecules and proteins but not to hyaluronan – a molecule that makes synovial fluid viscous.)

45 F T T T (NSAIDs cause salt and water retention and reduce renal blood flow disrupting renal autoregulation and GFR. Radiographic contrast media cause a transient decrease in GFR by an incompletely understood mechanism. Ranitidine has no effect on GFR.)

46 F T T T (It is a depolariser.)

47 F T T F (Placing an electromagnetic flow meter over the aorta is a very invasive procedure and is done only on animal models. Cardiac output is the Oxygen consumption divided by the A–V difference in the lungs.)

48 T T T F (Increase in stroke volume increases cardiac output and occurs in exercise.)

49 T T T T

50 F T T T (Pearson's coefficient of linear correlation is a parametric test.)

Paper 4 Answers

1 F F T T (Progression to AIDS is defined in the UK by the development of one of the AIDS-defining illnesses such as candidiasis (oesophageal and tracheal) CMV disease, lymphoma or Kaposi's sarcoma etc. About 85% of HIV/AIDS patients develop *Pneumocystis carinii* pneumonia.)

2 F T F T (BCG is the only live attenuated bacterial vaccine. Subunit vaccines are used for active immunisation, e.g. cholera.)

3 T F T F (Antiemetics may interact with opioid analgesics, NSAIDs and antihypertensives but not with local anaesthetics. Other drugs that interact with local anaesthetics are tricyclic antidepressants and sulphonamides. Hence, avoid local anaesthetic solutions or sprays in patients treated with co-trimoxazole.)

4 T F T F (It causes an increase in intracellular calcium. It takes 1–4 hours to achieve its peak effect even when given IV.)

5 T F T F (In late diastole the mitral and tricuspid valves are open. Blood flows into the heart filling the atria and ventricles throughout diastole.)

6 T T F T (Coagulopathics are uncommon in the first hour of trauma.)

7 F F T F (Hyperaldosteronism causes hypertension. Cushing's results in loss of muscle bulk of the limbs. Cardiovascular collapse occurs in the setting of hyposecretion of adrenocortical hormones.)

8 T T T T

9 F T T T (Koilonychia is most commonly seen in iron deficiency anaemia.)

10 T F T F (Glycoprotein IIb/IIIa complex is present in the platelet membrane. The damaged blood vessel undergoes a temporary reflex nervous vasoconstriction.)

11 F F T T (The ramus has a coronoid process. The foramen is on the ramus and not the body for the inferior dental nerve.)

12 F T T F (The auditory cortex lies in the upper part of the temporal lobe. Injury to the frontal lobes causes disinhibition.)

13 T T T F (The three tendons supporting the medial arch are tibialis anterior and posterior and flexor hallucis longus. Calcaneal fractures are typically caused by falls from heights landing on the feet.)

14 T T T T (Inclusion and exclusion criteria help us evaluate the external validity or applicability of the study.)

15 F T T F (Secondary closure is indicated when the skin edges are devitalised or when there is significant tissue loss which may cause undue tension if attempted to close or for a healing ulcer.)

16 F T F T (Antagonists reduce the effect of agonists by binding to the same sites on the receptor or to separate, but closely associated sites.)

17 T T F T (Tricyclics cause a sinus tachycardia.)

18 T T T F (Wet clothes conduct heat several hundred times as rapidly as air.)

19 T F T F (The pudendal canal is a space within the obturator fascia lining the lateral wall of the ischioanal fossa. It contains the pudendal nerve which is anaesthetised by local anaesthetic to relieve the pain of child birth. It also contains the pudendal artery, vein and the nerve to the obturator internus.)

20 F F F F (The thoracic wall has an ill-defined deep fascia. Its transverse diameter is increased by the elevation of the vertebrochondral ribs (7–10). It has seven pairs of typical ribs and five pairs of atypical ribs. The costochondral joints are primary cartilaginous joints.)

21 T F T T (The normal serum osmolality is between 275 and 295 mOsm/kg.)

22 T T F T (It is not as accurate as invasive methods such as arterial blood sample or central mixed venous saturation.)

23 T T T F (Red flags are possible indicators of serious spinal pathology. They include thoracic pain, fever and unexplained weight loss, bladder or bowel dysfunction, history of carcinoma, ill health or presence of other medical illness, progressive neurological deficit, disturbed gait, saddle anaesthesia, age of onset <20 years or >55 years.)

24 T T F T (Hepatitis A never progresses to chronic liver disease.)

25 T F T F (An LP is contraindicated if the patient has a reduced level of consciousness or focal neurological deficits. IV dexamethasone before antibiotics reduces mortality and neurological sequelae in pneumococcal meningitis.)

26 F T T T (The capitulum is the first secondary ossification centre to appear at about one year of age.)

27 F F T T (The appendix is suspended from the terminal ileum by the mesoappendix. It is derived from the midgut.)

28 T T T T (ABO antigens are present on lymphocytes but in much smaller amounts than on red cells.)

29 T T T F (It depresses erythropoiesis.)

30 T T T T

31 T T F F (It decreases protein breakdown to allow accumulation of protein in the cell. The hypothalamus secretes growth hormone releasing factor.)

32 T F T F (Renal compensation takes 48–72 hours for full effect. The PCO_2 is always raised in respiratory acidosis.)

33 F F F T (The Frank–Starling curves show the relationship between stroke volume and end-diastolic pressure. It is shifted to the right when contractility is increased. Transplanted hearts are denervated but obey the Frank–Starling principle and behave similar to a normal heart.)

34 T T T T (The incubation period is variable ranging from weeks to years and averages about 1–3 months. Fever, malaise and headache are followed by marked anxiety and agitation. Death occurs in 10–14 days. The vaccine is the human diploid cell vaccine – HDCV.)

35 T T F T (The middle cranial fossa lies over the roof of this cavity.)

36 F F F T (The vertebral artery does not pass through the foramen of C7 but starts at C6. C7 also does not have a bifid spine. Lateral flexion and nodding occur at the atlanto-occipital joint.)

37 T F T F (People perceive pain at almost the same degree of tissue damage. Burning pain stimulus travels along fibres that pass through the reticular substance of the brainstem and pain from pricking terminate in the vertebro-basal complex of the thalamus.)

38 F T F T (CSF is produced in the roof of the ventricles. The arachnoid granulations project into the superior sagittal sinus.)

39 F T F T (No single mechanism accounts for its therapeutic action although one minor mechanism is thought to be due to stimulation of the Na–K pump. It often is associated with nephrogenic diabetes insipidus.)

40 T T F F (Protamine binds to heparin and makes it unavailable to interact with proteins involved in formation of the blood clot.)

41 F T F T (Oliguria is defined as urine output less than 400 mL/day. Acute tubular necrosis causes severe hyperkalaemia.)

42 F F F T (The vital capacity is the sum of inspiratory reserve volume, tidal volume and the expiratory reserve volume. The residual volume cannot be measured with the spirometer. The FEV1/FVC ratio decreases in obstructive airways disease.)

43 T T F F (The aqueous humour is secreted in the posterior chamber and flows to the anterior chamber through the pupil. The macula has more cones than rods.)

44 T T F T (There are no sebaceous glands on the palms and soles.)

45 F T T T (The power of a study is the probability of correctly rejecting the null hypothesis when it is false.)

46 T T T T

47 T T T T

48 F T F F (Spontaneous retinal artery pulsation is an abnormal finding, which may occur if the intraocular pressure is very high or the central retinal artery pressure is very low. Spontaneous venous pulsation is frequently seen in normal eyes. Formation of capillary microaneurysms, seen as tiny red spots around the macula is a hallmark of diabetic retinopathy. The optic disc and surrounding retina are pale in central retinal artery occlusion.)

49 F F T F (It is the smaller of the two divisions and lies between extensor hallucis longus (EHL) and tibialis anterior just above the ankle joint and between EHL and extensor digitorum on the dorsum of the foot. It is rarely injured due to its deep location within the anterior compartment of the leg.)

50 F F F F (The anterior lobe is larger than the posterior. They are connected by pars intermedia. The body of the sphenoid bone lies below. Tumours do not affect visual acuity but visual fields.)

Paper 5 Answers

1 F F T T (It is uncommon for vaginitis to coexist with UTI. Patients with a UTI can have a low number of leucocytes in the urine, e.g. 6–20 per high-powered field and this may not be detected on dipstick.)

2 T T F F (A PUO is defined as a prolonged fever for over 3 weeks and resists diagnosis after a week in hospital. A subphrenic abscess is a well-known cause of a PUO. Other examples are pelvic abscess, empyema, TB, lymphomas, SLE and drugs.)

3 F F F F (The common iliac arteries arise in front of L4 body and bifurcate in front of the sacroiliac joints to their terminal branches the external and internal iliac arteries. They do not give visceral branches. They lie anterior and to the left of the internal iliac veins. The ureters cross anterior to the terminal bifurcation of the common iliac arteries.)

4 F F T T (The peripheral part of the intervertebral disc is called annulus fibrosus. Ligamentum flavum links the laminae.)

5 T T F T (In rheumatoid arthritis the most common type of anaemia is normocytic normochromic.)

6 T T T T

7 F T T T (Low or normal levels of C-reactive protein does not rule out inflammation or infection.)

8 F F F F (Rectal temperature is more by 0.6°C than the oral temperature. The anterior part of hypothalamus is responsible for heat loss. Increased thyroid hormone production occurs after prolonged exposure to cold, e.g. weeks. The body can produce 1.5 L of sweat per hour when excessively hot.)

9 T T F F (Primary hyperaldosteronism, i.e. Conn's syndrome causes hypernatraemia. Urine osmolality can be variable depending on the cause of hypernatraemia.)

10 F T T F (Only 1% of oxygen in the blood is carried in the dissolved state. Metabolic alkalosis increases the affinity of haemoglobin to oxygen.)

11 T F F T (Presents as right upper quadrant pain in women not men and is due to perihepatitis called Fitz Hugh and Curtis syndrome. It has a sensitivity of 90% but has many false-negative results. Recommended treatment is azithromycin 1 g oral once or doxycycline 100 mg BD for 7 days.)

12 F T T F (The auriculotemporal nerve supplies the scalp over the temporal region and anterior to the ear. Scalp lacerations bleed profusely because the vessels in the connective tissue are prevented from retracting.)

13 T F T F (The posterior mediastinum is traversed by the descending aorta, azygos and hemiazygos veins, vagus nerves, splanchnic nerves, lymph nodes, the thoracic duct and the oesophagus. It extends posteriorly down to the T12 vertebra level.)

14 F T T T (CSF protein levels are not related to serum or plasma protein levels. The normal range in adults is 0.15–0.45 g/L.)

15 T T T T

16 F T F F (Ketamine binds to NMDA receptors, increases ICP and more commonly causes nightmares in adults.)

17 T T T F (They inhibit a rise in intracellular cyclic GMP and hence decrease mediator release from mast cells.)

18 F F T T (The cardiac output is the product of the stroke volume and heart rate. $CO = SV \times HR$)

19 T F F T (In haemorrhagic shock there is increased secretion of vasopressin, glucagon, adrenaline, noradrenalin and aldosterone.)

20 F T F T (The phrenic nerve originates from C3 to C5 spinal levels. The caval opening in the diaphragm is T8 vertebral level.)

21 F T T F (The carpal tunnel is formed anteriorly at the wrist by a deep arch formed by the carpal bones and the flexor retinaculum. The median nerve is anterior to the tendons in the carpal tunnel.)

22 T T T T

23 F T F F (Males affected more often than females. Biopsy shows IgA deposition. Typically, recurrences of the clinical manifestations occur over a varying period lasting from a week to several months.)

24 T F F F (Exophthalmos is thought to occur because of the autoimmune mechanism and causes overgrowth of tissues retro-orbitally. So, it does not resolve with antithyroid treatments. Atrial fibrillation resolves with treatment of the underlying hyperthyroidism and cardioversion to sinus rhythm rarely works. Hyperthyroidism is most commonly caused by an autoimmune process.)

25 T T T T

26 T F F T (The vertebral artery lies on the posterior arch of the atlas vertebrae. The alar ligament is attached to the dens of the axis and the medial side of the occipital condyle.)

27 T T F F (Avulsion fractures occur due to sudden severe or repetitive stress applied to the muscle insertion at the bone. Avulsion fracture of the ischial tuberosity is caused by adductor magnus muscle attachment.)

28 T F T T (Testing of needle for presence of blood-borne viruses is not recommended.)

29 F T F T (Cysticercosis is caused by autoinfection or heteroinfection by eggs of *T. solium* and invasion of tissues by the intermediate larval form – cysticercus cellulosae. Hydatid cysts are caused by infection with hexacanth embryos of the dog tapeworm *Echinococcus granulosus*.)

30 T F T F (They are lipid-insoluble and hence do not enter living cells well. The difference is in the chemical structure of the drug nucleus.)

31 T T F F (Allopurinol inhibits drug metabolising enzymes. Chronic alcohol intake causes enzyme induction.)

32 F T T F (The respiratory centre is situated in the pons and medulla. The pneumotaxic centre switches inspiration off.)

33 T F T T (The elderly are especially deaf to high-frequency sounds.)

34 T T F T (Arteriovenous nipping is seen in hypertensive retinopathy.)

35 T T T F (McMurray test is used to assess meniscal injury.)

36 T F T T (A fall in pH decreases affinity of oxyhaemoglobin for oxygen. This is known as the Bohr effect. This enhances release of oxygen from haemoglobin in tissue capillaries where lower pH exists.)

37 T T T T

38 T T F T (It divides into the tibial and common peroneal nerves.)

39 F T T F (These tendons form the superomedial border. From superficial to deep it goes tibial nerve, popliteal vein and deepest the popliteal artery.)

40 T T F F (The external carotid artery terminates by dividing into the superficial temporal and maxillary arteries behind the neck of the mandible. It lies medial to the retromandibular vein and the facial nerve in the parotid gland.)

41 F T T F (Random sampling is the selection of people from a defined population of interest in such a way that each person has the same chance of being selected. Randomisation or random allocation is

between experimental and control groups and means that study participants are allocated to the groups in such a way that each has an equal chance of being in either group. The intervention or exposure is the independent variable.)

42 F F T T (The immature T lymphocytes arise in bone marrow and migrate to the thymus to complete maturation. T cells do not produce immunoglobulins. B cells produce immunoglobulins.)

43 F F T F (They work by blocking postsynaptic dopamine receptors. Chlorpromazine has more than 60 metabolites. They should not be used to treat withdrawal from other drugs as they may aggravate adverse reactions.)

44 F F T F (Insulin is a small protein hormone with a MW of 5808. It promotes glycogen storage in the liver and it reduces circulating free fatty acids by promoting triglyceride storage in adipocytes.)

45 F F T T (The hypothalamus secretes corticotrophin-releasing factor which stimulates the anterior pituitary to secrete ACTH. Glucocorticoids decrease utilisation of glucose by cells.)

46 T T F T (The manubriosternal joint is at T4 vertebral level.)

47 F F F F (The narrow folds are called folia. It consists of the two lateral cerebellar hemispheres and the median vermis. The middle pair connects it to the pons and not to the midbrain. The inferior aspect of the cerebellum is supplied by the posteroinferior cerebellar branch of the vertebral arteries.)

48 F T F F (Constriction is caused by contraction of the pupillary sphincter. About 1–1.5 mm is the smallest size of the pupil. Syphilis has a predilection for destroying the pretectal nuclei in the brainstem.)

49 F F T F (End-diastolic volume or pre-load is increased by stronger atrial contractions, increased venous tone, increased pumping action of the skeletal muscle and increased negative intrathoracic pressure. Standing, increased intrapericardial pressure and decreased ventricular compliance (following MI) decrease the pre-load.)

50 T F T F (Anisocoria – slight inequality in the size of pupils is observed frequently and may be of no pathological significance. Clubbing of fingers and toes was found almost universally, but it is now observed in less than 10% of patients. It primarily occurs in those patients who have an extended course of untreated IE.)

Paper 6 Answers

1 T F T T (Other systemic factors that delay wound healing are malnutrition, systemic malignancy and its treatment – chemotherapy and radiotherapy, haemorrhage, sepsis, venous and lymphoedema and immunosuppressant drugs.)

2 T T F T (It causes hypotension mainly due to marked peripheral vasodilatation.)

3 T T T T (The interaction between heparin and protamine is an example of chemical antagonism.)

4 T T F F (Rigors occur when the hypothalamic thermostat has been reset high and the body has to use heat-producing mechanisms to attain this. Once the thermostat is corrected back to normal the body uses heat-losing mechanisms to lower the body temperature, e.g. vasodilatation.)

5 T F F T (The cricothyroid membrane is situated just inferior to the thyroid cartilage, between the cricoid and the thyroid cartilage. The jugular venous pulse is measured in the internal jugular vein.)

6 F F T F (The lumbar arteries are posterior branches of the abdominal aorta. The testicular arteries arise anteriorly from the abdominal aorta. The aorta divides into the common iliac arteries.)

7 T F T F (Mineralocorticoid deficiency in Addison's disease causes hyperkalaemia. Calcium gluconate infusion counteracts the effects of hyperkalaemia but does not have any effect on the potassium concentration.)

8 F T T T (Type I respiratory failure has normal $PaCO_2$.)

9 F T F F (Only one antipyretic should be used at a time. Ceftriaxone is no longer first-line agent as it affects calcium and cefotaxime does not. Most children with a febrile illness are managed without the need for any blood tests. Urine collected by bags is often contaminated and is no longer advocated.)

10 T F T F (Subjecting gastric washings to culture and Ziehl–Nielsen staining has been replaced by fibreoptic bronchoscopy with washings from affected lobes subjected to culture and staining.

Sputum from suspected TB patients is cultured on Ogana or Lowenstein–Jensen medium for 4–6 weeks.)

11 F F T T (Osteomyelitis is an infection of the medullary cavity of a bone. In idiopathic disease the causative organism is usually *Staph aureus*. Infection is occasionally caused by fungi, viruses and parasites.)

12 F T F T (Abduction is initiated by supraspinatus. The rotator cuff is formed by the tendons of supraspinatus, infraspinatus, teres minor and subscapularis muscles.)

13 T F F F (The sympathetic motor cells lie within the lateral grey horns. The cranial parasympathetic outflow is along cranial nerves III, VII, IX and X. Sympathetic postganglionic terminals at the sweat glands release acetylcholine.)

14 T T F T (Blast crisis is not seen in chronic lymphocytic leukaemia. It is usually the cause of death in chronic granulocytic leukaemia.)

15 T T T T

16 T T T F (In AIDS there is depletion of $CD4^+$ helper T cells.)

17 F T T T (Cortisol decreases the quantity of protein in all tissues except the liver.)

18 F T T F (The Pacinian corpuscle is deep and the Meissner's corpuscles are also found in the lips and fingertips.)

19 F T T F (Refractory shock is not unique to haemorrhagic shock. It occurs in other forms of shock. Various positive feedback mechanisms such as severe central ischaemia leading to vasomotor and cardiac area depression in the brain cause vasodilatation and bradycardia resulting in further drop of BP leading to vicious circle.)

20 T T F T (Chronic carriers are individuals who excrete Salmonella for at least one year.)

21 F F F T (The femoral nerve arises from the anterior divisions of L2, 3 and 4 and breaks up in the femoral triangle into its branches. It supplies all three vasti muscles of the thigh.)

22 F T T F (Upper and lower compartments are formed by the articular disc. When dislocated bilaterally it presents with the mouth wide open and an inability to close it.)

23 T T T F (The system has no effect on nitrogen balance.)

24 T F T F (The utricle and saccule house the maculae. The crista ampullaris is within the ampulla of the semicircular canal. These structures transmit information to the cerebellum to help it predict future imbalance and therefore prevent imbalance altogether.)

25 T F T F (Increased anticholinergic effects with tricyclics or antiparkinsonian drugs. Thioridazine and quinidine may cause significant arrhythmias.)

26 F F T T (The optimal size is 2–5 μm. About 80–90% of the total dose is deposited in the mouth or pharynx.)

27 T T T F (The rate of the idioventricular rhythm is approximately 45 beats per minute in complete heart block. In an infranodal block the heart rate can be as low as 15 beats per minute causing cerebral ischaemia resulting in dizziness and fainting – Stokes–Adams syndrome.)

28 F T T T (A sinoatrial exit block is a feature of sick sinus syndrome. A right bundle branch block is seen in 1.5 per thousand population aged 20–40 years. A right axis deviation is seen in children and young thin adults. A Mobitz type 1 AV block is seen in athletes with high vagal tone.)

29 T F T F (The visceral afferent fibres return from T11 to L2 spinal levels and therefore the referred pain is from loin to groin. The renal pelvis lies posterior to the renal vessels.)

30 F F F T (The subclavian vein forms the brachiocephalic vein at the level of the sternoclavicular joint. The phrenic nerve lies behind the vein and in front of the artery.)

31 F F T T (The mean is a good measure of central tendency in normally distributed data. In skewed distribution, the median is better measure of the central tendency. The mean is lower than the median in negatively skewed distributions.)

32 F F F T (Prothrombin time is prolonged in deficiency of factors II, V, VII, X and fibrinogen. Activated partial thromboplastin time prolongation with normal prothrombin time usually indicates deficiency of either factor VIII or factor IX. Prolongation of thrombin time results from either hypofibrinogenaemia or from presence of inhibitors.)

33 F T F F (In quinsy the uvula is pushed to the opposite side of the affected tonsil. Acute laryngotracheobronchitis or croup is most commonly seen in the 1–2 year age group. Autophony is an abnormal perception of the patient's own voice. A sensation of sound in the absence of an appropriate auditory stimulus is called tinnitus.)

34 F T T T (Spontaneous respirations do not occur in brain stem death.)

35 T T T F (Aggregations of lymphoid tissue surround the nasopharyngeal region as the tubal, pharyngeal, palatine and lingual tonsils.)

36 F F F F (The manubriosteranal joint is a fibrocartilaginous or secondary cartilaginous joint. The costochondral joints are hyaline cartilaginous joints. The 11th and 12th ribs do not have tubercles and hence do not have costotransverse joints. The costovertebral and costotransverse joints are supplied by the thoracic dorsal rami.)

37 T F T F (Broad spectrum antibiotic use increases the risk of secondary fungal infections. Severe neutropenia is defined as an absolute neutrophil count of $<500/\text{mm}^3$.)

38 T T T F (Cryptogenic organising pneumonia is a pneumonia-like illness of unknown aetiology.)

39 T T F F (Aspirin overdose may cause hypothrombinaemia and inhibition of platelet aggregation but not thrombocytopenia.)

40 F T T F (Corticosteroids increase the neutrophil count in the peripheral blood.)

41 F F T F (The caudate controls gross movements. The putamen works in conjunction with the caudate nucleus. The subthalamic nucleus controls some aspects of the walking process.)

42 T T F F (In hypermetropia the light rays are not bent enough and therefore need correcting with a convex lens.)

43 F T F T (Intolerance to cold and weight gain are seen in hypothyroidism. Weight loss and intolerance to heat are features of hyperthyroidism.)

44 F T T F (Angina at rest is classed as Class 4 by the NYHA. Cushing's disease causes hypertension.)

45 T T F T (Pernicious anaemia is caused by vitamin B12 deficiency secondary to failure of secretion of intrinsic factor due to gastric atrophy.)

46 F F T T (Haemophilias are inherited as X-linked recessive disorder. The prothrombin time and bleeding time are normal and the activated partial thromboplastin time is prolonged.)

47 F T F T (The nerve to the obturator externus arises from the obturator nerve and does not exit from the lesser sciatic foramen. The inferior gluteal artery exits the pelvis through the greater sciatic foramen.)

48 T F T T (The geniohyoid and the thyrohyoid muscles are supplied by C1 fibres carried in the hypoglossal nerve. The interior mucosa is supplied by the internal laryngeal nerve over the vestibular fold including the sinus of the larynx.)

49 T T F T (The femoral nerve arises from L2, 3 and 4.)

50 T T F F (If the confidence interval crosses the line of zero difference then the results are not statistically significant. A tight confidence interval indicates a sample size that is large enough and that the value is probably close to the true value.)

Paper 7 Answers

1 T F T F (In the deoxygenated state the solubility of Hb-S is 10% than that of Hb-A. This leads to a conformational change in Hb-S causing the red cells to sickle. Haemoglobin Bart's is the most severe form of α-thalassaemia causing stillbirth or death within few hours of birth – hydrops fetalis.)

2 T F T F (Local treatment at bleeding site with pressure, topical haemostatics, immobilisation and appropriate wound management is effective in preventing prolonged bleeding and reducing need for replacement therapy. After administration of vitamin K correction of PT starts in 6 hours and can take up to 2 days to return to normal level.)

3 T F T F (The accessory duct opens just above the opening of the major duodenal papilla. The superior mesenteric vessels lie posterior to the neck of the pancreas.)

4 T T T F (Simple nasal bone fracture is a clinical diagnosis and routine radiography is unnecessary.)

5 F T T F (The long thoracic nerve arises from the anterior rami of C5–C7. The ulnar nerve is a terminal branch of the medial cord.)

6 T T F F (The null hypothesis is the opposite of the experimental or research hypothesis. The null hypothesis is that the independent variable does not affect the dependent variable in the manner proposed by the experimental hypothesis. In a positively skewed distribution the mean is higher than the median.)

7 F T F T (C3a and C5a increase vascular permeability but only C5a is chemotactic to most leucocytes. Nitric oxide inhibits platelet aggregation and adhesion.)

8 T T F T (Warfarin blocks the gama-carboxylation of several glutamate residues in prothrombin and factors VII, IX and X.)

9 F T T T (Ibuprofen is extensively metabolised in the liver and little is excreted unchanged.)

10 T F F T (They react with the receptor substance within the cytoplasm of the cell which then migrates to the nucleus where it activates specific genes. Growth hormone increases amino acid transport to all cells of the body.)

11 F F T F (It supplies ALL the muscles of the anterior compartment. It gives off a cutaneous branch which innervates the skin in the web space between the first and second toes and therefore does not need to be involved in a nerve block for anaesthesia of the sole.)

12 T F T F (The sacral outflow is S2, 3 and occasionally S4. Priapism is a clinical manifestation of injury to the sympathetic nervous system, i.e. priapism occurs due to unopposed parasympathetic activity.)

13 F F T T (An 'average' person weighing 70 kg contains about 42 L of water in total. The intracellular fluid compartment is twice as large as the extracellular compartment.)

14 T F F T (Minute volume is the product of respiratory rate and tidal volume. Lung compliance is the change in lung volume per unit change in pressure.)

15 T F T T (Occasionally, hypothyroidism occurs due to hypothalamic failure to secrete TSH.)

16 F T T F (Negri bodies are intracytoplasmic inclusion bodies found in hippocampal pyramidal cells and Purkinje cells in rabies. Polioviruses have propensity for the lower motor neurons in the anterior horns of the spinal cord.)

17 T F F T (50% of women may be asymptomatic. It is a Gram-negative diplococcus.)

18 F F T F (The two coronary arteries are the only branches of the ascending aorta. It is intrapericardial and is about 5 cm long ending at the level of the sternal angle of Louis. It is related posteriorly to the right main bronchus, right pulmonary artery and the left atrium both of which lie inferior to the left main bronchus.)

19 T F T F (A blow to the lower abdomen (steering wheel or seat belt) may cause a bladder injury without an associated pelvic fracture. The superior surface of the bladder is covered by peritoneum (and the upper part of the posterior surface in the male). It is separated from the pubic symphysis by loose areolar tissue.)

20 T F T T (Propylthiouracil and carbimazole induce severe neutropenia due to drug idiosyncrasy.)

21 F T T T (It is primarily a disease of the middle and old age, the majority of cases occurring between 40 and 80 years.)

22 T F T F (Antinuclear antibodies occur in other autoimmune disorders and in up to 10% of normal individuals. Anti-double-stranded DNA and anti-Smith antigen antibodies strongly suggest SLE. The kidneys are involved in virtually all cases of SLE.)

23 F F F T (The posterior pituitary stores these hormones but they are secreted by neuronal cells in the anterior hypothalamus. ADH is released in response to an increased concentration of sodium. ADH increases reabsorption of water in the collecting ducts not the tubules.)

24 T T T T (Inspiration accelerates heart rate while expiration decreases it. Increased activity in the atrial stretch receptors accelerates the heart.)

25 F T T F (Glucocorticoid used in endotoxin shock, a form of distributive shock is not effective in humans. Sudden autonomic activity results in vasodilatation and pooling of blood in veins leading to a faint. This occurs in neurogenic shock.)

26 F T T F (Folliculitis is an inflammation of the hair follicles and is confined to hair-bearing areas of the skin. Pseudomonas and herpes simplex are other less common causative organisms. The diagnosis is clinical and laboratory tests are rarely done.)

27 F F T T (It also consists of the amygdale. It is separated by the anterior limb.)

28 T F T F (Inversion/eversion occurs at the subtalar (talocalcaneal) joint. The anterior talofibular ligament is the most commonly injured.)

29 F F F T (They enter through the posterior roots. The first synapse is in the medulla. They traverse to the opposite side of the brainstem before going up further.)

30 F T T T (Decerebrate posturing suggests severe brain injury but not brain death which requires a GCS of 3.)

31 F T T T (Summation indicates the additive effect of two or more similarly acting drugs. Pharmaceutical interactions in vitro are responsible for loss of activity of a drug or their aggregation or precipitation in solution.)

32 F T F T (Glucagon is synthesised in the A cells of the islets of Langerhans. It has very potent inotropic and chronotropic effects on the heart.)

33 T T F F (They are called gamma but not delta fibres. The muscle spindle cannot contract but elongates when the end portions of the spindle contract so the CNS is apprised of the degree of elongation of the muscle spindle.)

34 T T T T (The premotor, the motor cortex together with the entire cerebellum and basal ganglia and the posture regulating system, corticospinal and corticobulbar systems take part in the planning and execution of voluntary movements.)

35 F F F T (The coronary sinus receives blood from the great cardiac vein, the posterior vein of the left ventricle, the middle cardiac vein, the small cardiac vein and oblique vein of the left atrium. It opens directly into the right atrium.)

36 T T F T (The palatine tonsil lies on the superior constrictor separating it from the facial artery and the carotid sheath.)

37 T T F T (Computerised random-number generators are an acceptable method of true randomisation and it eliminates any pseudo-randomisation.)

38 F F T T (The FAB classification is based on blood and bone marrow morphological features defined by Romanovsky and cytochemical staining. In this system acute lymphoblastic leukaemia is classified into three categories.)

39 T T T T

40 F F T T (There are more completed suicides in males than in females. People in the age group of <19 years and >45 years are at increased risk.)

41 T F T T (The VIth cranial nerve emerges at this junction.)

42 F T T T (The peritoneum covers the mesovarium and the anterior border of the ovary. The surface of the ovary is devoid of peritoneum and faces the peritoneal cavity.)

43 T F T F (The incubation period is usually 8–14 days and can be up to 21 days. A leucopoenia is a common finding on the FBC, and blood cultures should be done in the first week of the illness. Ciprofloxacin is the other first-line treatment with isolation and barrier nursing.)

44 F T T F (Giardiasis causes small intestinal disease with diarrhoea and malabsorption. Negative stool examination does not exclude the diagnosis as the parasite may be excreted at irregular intervals.)

45 T T F T (Hypokalaemia occurs due to aldosterone-like effect of corticosteroids.)

46 T F T T (It is spontaneously degraded by a process termed 'Hofmann degradation' and hence its elimination does not depend on either hepatic or renal function.)

47 T T T F (The heart rate increases by about 25 beats per minute when rising from the supine to the upright position. The drop in blood pressure is sensed by the carotid sinus and aortic arch which inhibits vagal tone in the medulla causing a reflex increase in heart rate.)

48 F F T T (The stapes stimulates the oval window. It is the thick basilar membrane that generates impulses.)

49 F T F T (A Gamekeeper's thumb is the rupture of the ulnar collateral ligament of the metacarpophalangeal joint. There is only one interphalangeal joint in the thumb. Kienbock's disease is an avascular necrosis of the lunate bone. Osteochondritis of the calcaneum is also known as Sever's disease.)

50 F F T F (See the following table for Glasgow Coma Scale score.)

Response	Score
Eye opening	
Spontaneous	4
To speech	3
To pain	2
None	1
Verbal response	
Orientated	5
Confused	4
Inappropriate words	3
Incomprehensible sounds	2
None	1
Best motor response	
Obeys commands	6
Localises pain	5
Withdrawal from pain	4
Flexion to pain	3
Extension to pain	2
None	1

Paper 8 Answers

1 F T T F (It is cyclic 3′,5′ adenosine monophosphate. It converts adenosine triphosphate to cyclic AMP.)

2 F T F T (ICP is normally 10 mm Hg.)

3 T F T T (A collapsing pulse is also seen in high fever, aortic regurgitation and AV fistulae. A jerky pulse is classical in HOCM. A slow rising pulse is seen in aortic stenosis. Pulsus paradoxus is seen also in massive pulmonary embolism, pericardial tamponade and constrictive pericarditis.)

4 T F F T (The serum K^+ is typically normal or high and the ABG should reflect a metabolic acidosis rather than a respiratory acidosis.)

5 T T F T (Cutaneous larva migrans is treated with either thiobendazole or ivermectin.)

6 T F F T (The median nerve innervates only the lateral two lumbricals. The cephalic vein originates from the lateral side of the dorsal venous arch.)

7 T T F F (Meckel's diverticulum is present in 2% of the population. The duodenojejunal flexure is surrounded by the ligament of Treitz.)

8 T T F F (Anion gap is the difference between the measured cations and anions. It represents the proteins in plasma. Normal gap is between 6 and 18 mmol/L. A high anion gap is found when bicarbonate is substituted with acids such as sulphuric, lactic or acetoacetate in various metabolic conditions.)

9 T T F F (Cushing's syndrome causes hypernatraemia. Sodium loss due to diarrhoea can be satisfactorily treated with oral therapy.)

10 T F T F (NSAIDs are the first choice of drugs in the treatment of acute gout. The alternative and second choice is colchicines, although there are no RCTs comparing colchicines with NSAIDs in matched patients.)

11 T F T T (Patients treated with sulphonylureas often gain weight exacerbating their resistance to insulin.)

12 T F T T (Rods provide black and white vision; the cones provide colour vision.)

13 T T T F (Tendons and ligaments can adapt to changes in their mechanical environment due to injury, disease or exercise.)

14 F F T T (The profunda brachii artery is the largest branch of the brachial artery. The common interosseous artery is a branch of the ulnar artery.)

15 F F T F (Right coronary artery occlusion results in an inferior infarction and involves the right ventricle in one third of inferior infarcts. Its posterior descending branch runs in the interventricular groove.)

16 T T F F (Positive predictive value is the proportion of those who test positive who actually have the disease. Negative predictive value is the proportion of those who test negative who do not have the disease.)

17 F T T F (A raised serum bilirubin and clinical jaundice are usual, but not invariable, in haemolytic anaemia. Spherocytosis occurs in a number of haemolytic anaemias of different aetiology and is not specifically diagnostic of any particular type of haemolytic anaemia.)

18 T F T F (Gigantism almost always occurs due to a GH-secreting acidophilic tumour of the pituitary. Acromegaly does not affect the growth of the sternum.)

19 T F F T (The Research Ethics Committee as well as the Clinical Ethics Committee have lay members along with professional medical and nursing members. A wrong diagnosis is not necessarily negligent as long as the appropriate standard of care was given to the patient.)

20 T F T T (The levator palpebrae superioris inserts into the eyelid and not the eyeball.)

21 F T F F (When the puboprostatic ligaments are transected in a pubic symphysis diastasis/fracture, the prostate gland 'rides high' and is not palpable on PR examination. The gland lies on the levator ani and its apex is against the superior fascia of the urogenital diaphragm. It is traversed by the ejaculatory ducts, formed by the union of the vasa deferentia and the seminal vesicles.)

22 T F T F (At least three films should be examined before malaria is declared unlikely. The thick films have a higher yield in diagnosis. There is wide spread resistance of *P. falciparum* to chloroquine.)

23 T T T F (Because of its often insidious onset, the fact that many patients are not known to have an abnormal valve or congenital heart lesion and pathognomonic signs of infective endocarditis e.g. splinter haemorrhages, Osler's nodes are rare the diagnosis is often delayed.)

24 T T T F (Drug interactions can be the result of pharmacokinetic, pharmacodynamic or a combination of these mechanisms. Some important drug interactions occur as a result of two or more mechanisms.)

25 F T F T (Diclofenac is a simple phenylacetic acid derivative that is a relatively non-selective cyclo-oxygenase inhibitor. Renal dysfunction does not influence clearance significantly.)

26 F F T T (Chorea is due to damage to the caudate nucleus and putamen. Athetosis is characterised by slow writhing movements of the peripheral parts of the body. Jumping from one movement pattern to another occurs in chorea.)

27 F T F F (The vasomotor centre is the most important area in the medulla that controls blood pressure. Baroreceptors in the aortic arch monitoring the arterial circulation sense a drop in BP and send impulses to the VMC to increase its activity, increasing BP. In hyperaldosteronism there is failure to increase BP when intrathoracic pressure returns to normal. Exposure to high concentration of CO_2 is associated with cutaneous and cerebral vasodilatation, with vasoconstriction elsewhere resulting in a slow rise in BP.)

28 F T T F (Direct inguinal hernias rarely strangulate. A saphena varix is a varicosity of the long saphenous vein at the site of the saphenous opening. This has a fluid thrill when the patient coughs due to an incompetent valve at the saphenofemoral junction.)

29 T F T F (Fournier's gangrene is an acute inflammatory oedema of the scrotum followed by sloughing gangrene. Erythema ab igne is the skin discolouration seen after applications of hot water bottles in attempts to relieve unremitting chronic pain.)

30 F T T T (Reed–Sternberg cells are large and are either multinucleated or have a bilobed nucleus – resembling an owl's eye appearance, with prominent eosinophilic nucleoli.)

31 F T T F (Factors II, VII, IX and X are vitamin K-dependent coagulation factors. In the intrinsic pathway the factor Xa is formed by activation of factor X by factor IXa.)

32 F T T F (The fallopian tube lymph drainage is to the pre-aortic and lateral aortic nodes. The anal canal below the pectinate line – transition zone between squamous and columnar epithelium, drains to the superficial inguinal nodes while that above the line drains to the internal iliac nodes.)

33 T T T T

34 T F T T (The internal intercostal muscles run downwards and backwards reaching the angle of the ribs.)

35 F T F T (Average or mean and median are measures of central tendency.)

36 T F T T (Acute cellular rejection responds promptly to immunosuppressive drugs.)

37 T T F F (The early features of systemic toxicity are numbness or tingling of the tongue or lips, light-headedness, anxiety and tinnitus. Convulsions and arrhythmias generally occur after this. The least toxic is prilocaine.)

38 F F T T (They reduce the hypersensitivity of the airways. There is no need to taper a 5-day course of oral prednisolone and should simply be discontinued at this point.)

39 F T T F (It is secreted mainly by zona glomerulosa. It causes only a small increase in cardiac output.)

40 F F T F (The piriformis muscle is an anatomical landmark in the pelvis. It is attached to the greater trochanter and exits through the greater sciatic foramen. The sciatic nerve emerges inferior to its lower border.)

41 T T F F (The lateral cutaneous nerve of the thigh arises directly from the lumbar plexus. The femoral nerve is easily blocked with local anaesthetics but only occasionally provides pain relief for patients with fractured neck of femur as the hip joint is also supplied by the obturator and sciatic nerves.)

42 F F T F (Osmolarity is the number of osmoles per litre of solution and osmolality the number per kilogram of solvent. Urinary osmolarity is not feasible because of the considerable variation in concentration of different solutes. Urinary osmolality should therefore be measured.)

43 T T T T

44 F F T F (In the corneal reflex the afferent limb is the trigeminal nerve and the efferent limb is the facial nerve. Bell's phenomenon is the upward rotation of the eyeball on trying to contract the weak orbicularis oculi. This is seen in lower motor neuron lesions of the facial nerve. The glossopharyngeal (IX) and vagus (X) nerves are the afferent and efferent limbs, respectively in the gag reflex.)

45 T F T F (The incubation period is 1–3 weeks. It is the commonest cause of epididymitis in men under the age of 35.)

46 F T T T (The cruciates take their name from their tibial origin.)

47 F T F T (The structures passing between the ureter and the pelvic peritoneum are the vas deferens in the male and uterine artery in the female. The obturator nerve is lateral to the ureter and the superior vesicle artery runs posterior to the ureter.)

48 F T F F (Epistaxis is the most common symptom and usually the presenting manifestation. The platelet count is usually normal. The skin lesions are seen mainly on the face, hand and feet.)

49 T F F F (The lifespan of platelets in circulation is about 8–10 days. The normal count ranges from 150 to 400 × 10^9/L. Platelets are anucleate, terminal stage of development of the megakaryocytic series.)

50 F F T T (Exudate is an inflammatory extravascular fluid with high protein concentration, high cellular debris and a specific gravity above 1.020. The intravascular osmotic pressure during acute inflammation is reduced due to leakage of high protein fluid.)